Praise for

"Having worked with Dr Yvonne Waft when training mental health professionals, and also knowing some of her life story, I knew her book would be good, and I agreed willingly to write a comment. My goodness, Yvonne even surpassed my expectations! I like this book so much because it explains in understandable language what trauma actually is, and gives tried and tested strategies to cope. Yvonne's book quite rightly sees trauma ranging from the small emotionally uncomfortable experiences that are drip-fed to so many of us growing up, to the big life-altering events which continue to impact us years later. For someone suffering the results of psychological trauma, Yvonne gives you strategies which work to help you manage and cope with life as it is for you now. These strategies will be particularly helpful if you haven't yet engaged in psychological therapy with a skilled professional, or you are on a long list awaiting a first appointment with services. From my perspective as someone who delivers psychological therapies, I would have valued reading this as an undergraduate psychologist, and again as a postgraduate in clinical psychology training, when I was trying to get to grips with how trauma impacts people. In addition to those early in their therapeutic career path, there is another group who I feel could benefit from reading this book – other professionals delivering psychological therapy who don't fully understand the way trauma impacts our brain and body, and who are humble enough to admit that to themselves."

Dr Michael C Paterson OBE
PhD DClinPsych CPsychol AFBPsS
Consultant Clinical Psychologist

"The author has written a raw and honest account of their own trauma experiences and how these have impacted not just at the time, but on their life journey and how they currently deal with life. This is the first time I have seen such a clear account of how an author's trauma has then been described from the perspective of them as a psychologist, to help us understand the impact. The impact is described in both psychological terms, but also how it effects the bodily reactions, physiology, neurological development. It allows the reader to really understand the context in which those who have experienced trauma are having to live in terms of their psychological responses and also how their nervous system has been impacted.

This book would be helpful for those who have experienced trauma who want to understand the impact is has had. It allows an in-depth understanding of how events in the past have affected people – it gives the science behind it, which allows a deep understanding and therefore allows multiple ways to help someone as they can see exactly why they feel the way they do and have the reactions they do. It also gives so many useful ways to help move on, manage and live a good life despite past experiences. The science behind the way to recover, allows the reader to not feel overwhelmed, but to give a context to how they feel and how to manage their difficult emotions.

The book gives a unique insight into the trauma experienced by someone who went on to become a skilled clinical psychologist. The author is able to use their extensive therapeutic training to understand how their experiences impacted them. Sharing this in the book means that the science comes to life and is relatable and easy to understand.

The book contains many ways forward for those who have had difficult experiences.

The book will be invaluable for mental health professionals working with people who have experienced trauma. Its easy language and lack of jargon makes it accessible and offers clear ways of helping people and explaining to our clients the impact their trauma has had.

It's written in a kind, compassionate and clear way.

The book is one of a kind in the field – a unique combination of the author's honest account of their trauma, written from their current perspective as an experienced psychologist. This allows the book to bring to life the theory we know about trauma but relating it to real life experiences.

The section of neurodiversity and trauma is particularly interesting and it allows us to understand the layers of trauma and the different impact it has on different people.

The book is uplifting and hopeful in that by understanding trauma responses in terms of the mind and body, the reader is able to fully understand how to heal and live their life.

It was a privilege to read such an honest account."

Dr Susan van Genderen
Consultant Clinical Psychologist
Director of Therapies
Black Country Healthcare NHS Trust

Coping with Trauma

Coping with Trauma

Surviving and thriving in the face
of overwhelming events

Dr Yvonne Waft

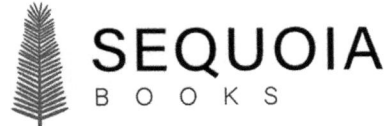

Every possible effort has been made to ensure that the information contained in this book is accurate at the time of going to press. The publishers and author(s) cannot accept responsibility for any errors and omissions, however caused. No responsibility for loss or damage occasioned to any person acting, or refraining from action, as a result of the material contained in this publication can be accepted by the editor, the publisher or the author.

First published in 2023 by Sequoia Books

Apart from fair dealing for the purposes of research or private study, or criticism or review, as permitted under the Copyright, Designs and Patents act 1988, this publication may only be reproduced, stored or transmitted, in any form or by any means, with the prior permission in writing of the publisher, or in the case of reprographic reproduction in accordance with the terms and licenses issued by the CLA. Enquiries concerning reproduction outside these terms should be sent to the publisher using the details on the website www.sequoia-books.com

©Yvonne Waft 2023

The right of Dr Yvonne Waft to be identified as author of this work has been asserted in accordance with the Copyright, Designs and Patents act 1988.

ISBN
Print: 9781914110306
EPUB: 9781914110313

A CIP record for this book is available from the British Library

Library of Congress Cataloguing-In-Publication Data

Name: Dr Yvonne Waft
Title: Coping With Trauma / Dr Yvonne Waft
Description: 1st Edition, Sequoia Books UK 2023
Print: 9781914110306
EPUB: 9781914110313

Library of Congress Control Number: 2023919441

Print and Electronic production managed by Deanta Global

In loving memory of my dear friend Sue who was as determined as I was that I should complete this book. Her own traumatic journey through leukaemia sadly ended as I worked on the final edits.

Susan Whitfield 2 February 1986 to 14 July 2023.

Fly high my beautiful friend.

Contents

Figures — xi
Foreword — xii
The Unique Perspective — xiii
Acknowledgements — xiv

Part One

1. What Do We Mean by "Trauma"? — 3
2. My Story — 13
3. Types of Trauma — 21
4. Impact of Trauma — 31
5. Added Complexity — 41
6. Trauma and the Brain — 52
7. Trauma and the Body — 63

Part Two

8. The Healing Journey — 75
9. Helpful vs Unhelpful Coping — 85
10. Resources for Healing — 94
11. Acceptance and Commitment Therapy — 103
12. Mindfulness — 111

13 Grounding/Getting Present   120
14 Dealing with Thoughts   129
15 Valued Living and Thriving   139
16 Conclusions and Further Help   148

Appendices: Worksheets and Questionnaires   159
References   170

Figures

4.1	The ACE Questionnaire. Source: Adapted from Shapiro (1990; revised 2021)	33
4.2	The ACE Pyramid. Source: Centre for Disease Control (CDC)	35
8.1	Maslow's Hierarchy of Needs	79
8.2	A-C-E Pie Chart	81
10.1	Diagram of Window of Tolerance. Source: Adapted from Siegal, 2002	96
10.2	Polyvagal Theory: The Autonomic Ladder. Source: Adapted from Dana D, 2018	98

Foreword

Dr Sarah Swan
Coping With – Series Editor
Consultant Clinical Psychologist

When I was diagnosed with breast cancer in 2019, I knew I was going to have to use my skills as a clinical psychologist to help me cope with the distress that this inevitably caused. Early on in my journey, I had the urge to write, as a way of processing my experiences. I immediately thought it had the potential for a book, but never thought this would come to fruition. But with the support of the Association of Clinical Psychologists, Sequoia Publishing, friends, family and colleagues, I committed to writing the book.

I began to realise what a unique position I held; facing a difficult life event that many others face, but with the knowledge and experience of a long career in helping people with their emotional experiences. Suddenly, it dawned on me that there could be any number of difficult or challenging experiences that other Clinical Psychologists may have faced. And, like me, they would in all likelihood have valuable skills to share with others facing the same situation. And so, the idea for the series was born.

It is an honour to launch the series with my book *Coping with Breast Cancer*. And it has been my pleasure to support other Clinical Psychologists with their writing in order to produce a series of books that will help to bring valuable psychological ideas to a wide audience. With the knowledge and skills of the writers, I am confident that this series will benefit many people facing difficult and challenging situations and give them helpful skills to cope.

The Unique Perspective

Dr Penelope Cream
Clinical and Health Psychologist
Director of Operations, ACP-UK

The Association of Clinical Psychologists (ACP-UK) is delighted to be publishing these important *Coping With…* books. In these pages, clinical psychologists have taken the courageous step of sharing how they applied their skills to their own lives, in order to help others facing similar difficulties and challenges.

The profession of clinical psychology spans many types of psychological approaches across all areas of the lifespan and of individual experiences, from physical health, psychological distress and mental illness, as well as cognitive difficulties, family challenges and workplace problems. Clinical psychologists have rigorous training not only in psychological therapies but also in research methods and using evidence-based practice. They draw on these aspects to inform everything they do, including looking after themselves. These books evidence the flexibility and creativity with which we can use and apply our skills, both to help ourselves and others.

It is not often that clinicians share their first-hand experiences of challenging situations and how they have applied what they have learnt in their training and the many years of experience that follow. I feel very proud of my clinical psychology colleagues who have written this series of books, not only for everything that they have experienced with courage and insight but for the generosity and openness with which they want to help other people. It is not easy to combine subjective personal experience with an external clinical perspective, yet in these books they share the breadth of knowledge and training that the profession brings us.

Acknowledgements

I am very grateful to the Association of Clinical Psychologists (ACP-UK) for creating the opportunity and the pathway for me to publish this book. This is something I have wanted to write for a long time, but without the support of the ACP, in particular Dr Penelope Cream and Dr Sarah Swan, I could not have envisaged having the time or opportunity to see this project through to publication. I especially want to acknowledge Dr Sarah Swan's helpful suggestions on the text, to ensure it is as clear and helpful as can be. I wish to acknowledge the contributions of all the many people I have learnt from throughout my career, tutors, supervisors, colleagues, but most of all the people who have come to me for therapy and taught me so much about trauma and its many impacts on us. I would like to acknowledge the encouragement I received early in my psychology career from Dr Pippa Dell (University of East London) and Dr Dave Green (University of Leeds) for their faith in my academic skills, which far outweighed my own confidence, had I listened to them this book may have been written many years earlier. Finally, this book could not have been written without the loving support of my husband, Bob, and daughter, Georgina, who have been very patient and supportive throughout the writing process, even when it has meant me going away for a few days to write in peace! Thank you everyone.

Part One

Part One

1 What Do We Mean by "Trauma"?

Introduction

The short answer to "What is Trauma?" is any overwhelming event that a person experiences, where they are powerless to deal effectively with the situation. This can have devastating and, often, long-term consequences for the person and for those around them. Obvious examples would be experiences in combat zones, natural disasters, severe assaults and accidents. Less obvious examples would be captivity, childhood neglect and abuse, controlling and coercive relationships, any form of hatred or discrimination, poverty and deprivation.

Since the late 1980s/early 1990s, our understanding of the impact of psychological trauma on human beings has begun to be understood far better than ever before. Psychologists and neuroscientists have developed new ways of understanding what goes on in the human mind and body when overwhelming events occur, and from this understanding have come new ways of helping people to deal with the aftereffects of trauma. My aim in this book is to distil as much of that new learning as I can into a helpful format to enable those living with the aftereffects of trauma to cope better with what has happened to them and find ways to live their best lives. I hope to dispel a few myths along the way and provide the reader with tools they can use in everyday life to help stabilise emotions and live life to their full potential.

The first myth to be dispelled is that we humans were born to be happy. If you believe everything the advertising industry tries to tell you, you imagine that if you just had the right house, the right furniture, the right car, clothes, perfume, make-up and so on, you too could be as happy as the people portrayed in the commercials. However, humans did not evolve to be happy, contented, fulfilled beings! Like all animals, we evolved to survive and reproduce, to pass on our genes to the next generation in an endless cycle. Our early ancestors grew up in times of great hardship, without modern conveniences such as electricity, medicine or mobile phones. If you think about it, in survival terms, we are in fact fairly rubbish animals! We don't have the teeth and claws of the great predators, and we don't have the speed and agility of prey animals such as the antelope, monkeys or the squirrels in my garden. We cannot outrun a cheetah or swing effortlessly up into the treetops away from danger. We are, in fact, very vulnerable creatures, and our ancient ancestors had to deal with many very real threats to their survival. Fortunately for us humans though, the majority of us have pretty good intellect and communication skills and that is what enabled our ancestors to survive and evolve to be the highly successful species we believe ourselves to be today, despite the many traumas our ancestors faced in their daily lives.

It is our intellect that has allowed us to perceive and predict threats to our survival and invent increasingly complex solutions to overcome these. Our communication skills have enabled us to band together in social groups to face down predators and marauding tribes and to tell stories so that our children and their children in turn can learn the lessons of survival. Our ancestors learnt to work together and communicate with each other to solve the problems of feeding their families, protecting their homes, warding off predators, conquering lands and building civilisations to maximise the survival potential of their tribes. It is thanks to these higher-order thinking skills that civilisations were developed, that science and medicine and technology have grown. It is also thanks to these higher-order thinking skills that we are all extremely good at imagining problems and threats and worrying ourselves silly about possible solutions and outcomes. In many ways, our success as a species is also our downfall!

A Brief History of Trauma Studies

The study of psychological trauma has gone in and out of fashion since at least the late nineteenth century and has a rather chequered history. Herman (1992) describes this as beginning with a Parisian Neurologist, Jean-Martin Charcot, in the late 1800s. Charcot ran a large asylum, called the Salpêtrière, on the banks of the river Seine in Paris. This hospital had been established in the seventeenth century as an asylum for elderly, infirm and insane women. Charcot studied neurology and psychiatry, and many aspiring physicians studied under his supervision, including most famously, Sigmund Freud. Charcot and his many disciples were all keen to understand the causes of 'hysteria', a predominantly female condition that had baffled the exclusively male, medical establishment for centuries. Hysteria was a broad term encompassing many emotional, psychological and physical symptoms including altered states of consciousness, mood disturbances, paralysis, loss of feeling in the body, convulsions and amnesia. Having studied under Charcot, Freud returned to his home city of Vienna and set up a clinic treating hysterical middle-class women. Based on what those women revealed through their work with him, Freud soon concluded that hysteria was a condition caused by psychological trauma, the memories of which had been suppressed or forgotten somehow. He asserted that uncovering the lost memories through psychoanalysis, putting them into words and releasing the intense feelings that accompany the memory could heal the hysterical symptoms (Herman, 1992). Freud went further and concluded in his 1896 paper 'The Aetiology of Hysteria' that every case of hysteria had its origins in the trauma of early sexual abuse (Freud, 1896). His thesis, not surprisingly, proved unpopular in the reserved upper middle classes of Vienna where he practiced. Rather than face being ostracised by the very people who made up his clientele, he subtly changed his conclusion to say that it was merely female fantasy that led to hysteria and that their reports of actual sexual abuse were simply untrue. Effectively what this did for the next hundred years or so was to blame women for their dirty minds and for the neuroses that stemmed from their impure thoughts. With Freud's abrupt about-turn, the study of psychological trauma was sadly put on pause for several decades.

The study of psychological trauma and hysterical conditions has then taken on new energy with each major war. The two world wars of the first half of the twentieth century provided many new cases of neurosis, resembling 'hysteria', but this time it was in men exposed to the horrors of trench warfare. 'Hysteria' was by its very definition a female issue as the term comes from the Greek word for womb. A new diagnosis was needed for men showing the same symptoms. The notion of 'shell-shock' was initially put forward, suggesting that the neurotic symptoms were caused by the physical trauma of being in close proximity to artillery explosions. Inconveniently for this theory, the same condition was also seen in men who had not been exposed to such physical trauma, and a conclusion was reached that perhaps it was the prolonged exposure to violence and death that underpinned the condition. This then begged the question of whether warfare was to blame, or whether it was just the weak moral fibre of certain men that meant they could not cope with it. Rather like Freud's female clients, the blame was then laid squarely on the victim for their moral failings. Victim blame is another myth I would very much like to dispel throughout this book. Is it really a weakness to be greatly upset by witnessing death and destruction in war?

The Vietnam War in the 1970s created a further opportunity to study the effects of trauma on humans. Many Vietnam veterans returned home to the United States with symptoms similar to 'hysteria' and 'shell-shock', adding weight to the theory that there is something that happens when people are exposed to extreme events that leads to a consistent set of highly distressing symptoms. This led finally to a recognition of one rather obvious fact, that traumatic events cause intense distress, that is, when bad things happen, people are frequently left very upset and disturbed, and there is a consistent pattern to how this manifests.

Also, around the mid-1970s, more and more women were able to access higher education. There was a growth in women's studies and the feminist movement both in the United Kingdom and the United States. From these studies came a confirmation of Freud's original proposition that sexual abuse of women and children was rife and that the trauma this causes has lasting effects on women's health, both physically and mentally. Herman (1992) reports on a study in the 1980s by sociologist Diana Russell, which found that in a random sample of 900 women, one in four had been raped and one in three had been sexually abused in childhood. She goes on to state,

> *Only after 1980, when the efforts of combat veterans had legitimated the concept of post-traumatic stress disorder, did it become clear that the psychological syndrome seen in survivors of rape, domestic battery and incest was essentially the same as the syndrome seen in survivors of war. The implications of this insight are as horrifying in the present as they were a century ago: the subordinate condition of women is maintained and enforced by the hidden violence of men. There is a war between the sexes. Rape victims, battered women, and sexually abused children are its casualties. Hysteria is the combat neurosis of the sex war.* Herman (1992) p32.

I would argue that news reports of violence against women and children in the early 2020s in the UK show that not much has changed in the intervening decades.

Post-Traumatic Stress Disorder

Almost a hundred years after Freud first put forward the idea that traumatic events cause mental distress, debates around the returning Vietnam veterans and their mental disturbances finally led to the American Psychiatric Association adding post-traumatic stress disorder (PTSD) to its manual of mental disorders in 1980. They acknowledged that threats to our survival and our responses to them underlie a consistent set of difficulties in the traumatised person. In the most recent iteration of the manual, DSM-5 Diagnostic and Statistical Manual (the clinician's guide to difficulties and diversity within the human mind and brain) a traumatic event is defined as *"exposure to actual or threatened death or serious injury, or sexual assault"* (American Psychiatric Association, 2022). This means that events which threaten one's survival, or the survival of one's closest allies, are considered traumatic and can cause a range of unpleasant experiences. If these meet certain criteria, they can then be diagnosed as PTSD. The criteria have been modified somewhat since the first iteration of the disorder in DSM 3 (DSM 3, 1980), but the main features recognised since the 1980s are as follows:

1. **'Intrusion Symptoms'** such as unwanted thoughts, images, emotions and body sensations. This would include flashbacks, where a person vividly re-experiences aspects of the disturbing event as if it was actually happening again, and nightmares.
2. **'Avoidance Symptoms'** such as avoiding thoughts and feelings about the disturbing event by using distraction techniques, using alcohol or drugs, keeping extremely busy and refusing to talk about the disturbing event, and avoiding external reminders of the disturbing event such as certain people, places and situations.
3. **'Mood and Cognition Symptoms'** such as anxiety, low mood, negative beliefs about the self and strong emotions such as fear, horror, anger, guilt or shame.
4. **'Hyperarousal Symptoms'** such as irritability, angry outbursts, jumpiness, poor sleep, inability to relax and hyper-vigilance.

Diagnostic Controversy

The question of whether this should really be considered a 'disorder' or whether it is simply a healthy adaptation to bad stuff happening is the subject of much debate among experts. From a medical model perspective, people who seem different, physically and/or mentally, are seen as sick and in need of medical treatment to facilitate a return to the norm. Whereas, a more social model would see the problem as being located in society and the experiences a person has had (see, for example, Oliver, 1996). Within psychology, there is a view that most, if not all, mental distress can be explained in terms of the experiences people have been subjected to at a personal, familial and societal level.

The Power, Threat, Meaning Framework (PTMF) is proposed by some psychologists as an alternative to the medical model of mental distress (Johnstone et al, 2018). Very briefly, rather than focusing on what might be medically wrong with a mentally distressed person, the PTMF focuses more on what has happened to the person to cause the distress. The PTMF encourages clinicians to consider the ways in which power has operated in a person's life in the form of race, wealth, age, ability, sexuality, gender and so on. Then from there, look at the threats that have been posed to the person, such as racism, ableism, violence and poverty. From there, we can look at the meaning the person has made from those experiences, recognising that there will be much crossover between characteristics and each person's unique profile which will lead to unique outcomes.

It is tempting to become polarised in our viewpoints on issues around diagnosis. Is PTSD a valid diagnosis of a disorder, or is it simply a description of how someone typically behaves when they have been through extreme events? Personally, I prefer to hold both extremes lightly. If it is useful to a person to see their difficulties in terms of a medical diagnosis, then who am I to stop them? If someone prefers to think of their distress as a very valid response to abnormal circumstances, then I'm all for supporting them in that too. Where I really want to be helpful as a psychologist is in helping to reduce the distress where I can. What we do know is that people who have experienced a significant amount of bad stuff in their lives can struggle with a wide range of difficulties. When I work therapeutically with a person, I care very little about whether they meet the diagnostic criteria for any particular disorder. Rather, I try to understand what they have been through and how they have tried to cope, and then we work together to find new ways of coping that I hope may serve them better in the future.

In the first half of this book, I aim to explore with you in more detail what psychological trauma is, the different types of psychological trauma and how it manifests in the mind and body. This is important because half the battle is to realise that post-traumatic stress, however it manifests, is a normal reaction to abnormal, overwhelming circumstances. Understanding the mechanisms at work, and why we have them, helps to reassure us that we are not going mad, we are not failing, we are not weak, and we are certainly not to blame for what is happening. We are simply doing the best we can, with what resources we have at the time, to cope with the overwhelming experiences. Then, in the second half of the book I will explore what strategies can help us to manage the difficulties that develop when significant trauma has been a feature of our lives, and when we might need additional help to move on from traumatic events.

I shall be exploring this complex field with you from two perspectives. First, I am a UK-registered Clinical Psychologist with many years of experience working and studying in the field of trauma assessment and trauma therapy. I have learnt to assess psychological trauma in the very formal context of legal assessments for Personal Injury and Medical Negligence claims. I have worked therapeutically with many hundreds of people within the NHS in the UK, and also, in Private Practice in the UK, most of whom have experienced significant trauma in their lives. Second, I also write this book from the perspective of a human being who has lived through considerable trauma in my own life and will share reflections of my own very real experiences of trauma, its aftermath and its healing.

I came into clinical psychology in the mid-1990s, shortly after the first edition of Judith Herman's important book *Trauma and Recovery* was published. Over the course of my career, I have seen tremendous growth in the understanding and acceptance of trauma and its consequences as a legitimate area of study. With the advent of brain-scanning technologies since the latter part of the twentieth century, neuroscientists have been able to see in real time what happens in human brains when traumatic material is presented to them, or when they are reminded of their own traumatic events. We now have a much better understanding of the neurobiology of trauma. Alongside this development, new treatments for trauma symptoms have been developed which can transform lives. The study of trauma therapy has led to an understanding of the pervasiveness of trauma in society. It is not just sexual trauma and warfare that cause people to suffer, although these are very prevalent issues. People can be traumatised by inadequate parenting, bullying and assault of all kinds, accidents, illnesses, bereavements and natural disasters too.

Writing about trauma is almost inevitably going to mean discussing issues that some people may find difficult to read. For the most part, I will not be describing other people's traumatic events that I have heard about in therapy in any detail as there is a risk that I could breach someone's confidentiality so the majority of my descriptions will be much more generic in nature, and I will invent some composite characters to illustrate the kinds of experiences real people report in research and therapy. In doing this, I will need to allude to themes that some people will find troubling, and this is unavoidable in a book of this nature. As we will learn, avoiding traumatic material can exacerbate our difficulties with it, and confronting it, although painful, can ultimately help us to resolve it. When my daughter was little, we had a copy of Michael Rosen's children's book *We're Going on a Bear Hunt*. In each section of the Bear Hunt, the family comes across an obstacle such as 'long, wavy grass' or a 'deep, cold river' and each time there is the phrase 'we can't go over it, we can't go under it, oh, no, we've got to go through it'. I often use this as an analogy for dealing with trauma. In therapy, when we want to get past a traumatic memory, we can't go over it, we can't go under it, oh, no, we've got to go through it! While this book may at times bring up painful feelings for you, I would see this as part of the process of healing, starting to recognise and confront whatever you have been through. I would add though, you must take it at your own pace, give yourself time to notice your own responses to the material and respond to yourself with compassion and patience. I will be providing exercises and helpful skills that you can practice to make this process easier, so take the time and go gently through this book. It is important to state that a self-help guide alone may not be sufficient to resolve your own trauma experiences, and you may find as you read this book that you feel a need to seek out professional help for your difficulties. Towards the end of the book, I will provide some guidance on finding appropriate help as it can be difficult to find good quality therapy and support for trauma-related difficulties, and the field of psychological therapy is not very well regulated in many parts of the world.

Chapter Summary

- From Freud and Charcot attempting to understand hysteria in the late 1800s through Judith Herman's seminal book in the early 1990s, to our present understanding, trauma theory has taken many turns and developed exponentially, sometimes right back to where it started!
- Knowledge and understanding of trauma have been aided by war, feminist research and the advent of neuroscience and brain-scanning technology.
- The more we know, the more we don't know! With the recognition of PTSD as a medical disorder in 1980, a new debate emerged around the notion of disorder versus the idea that trauma is a normal reaction to abnormal circumstances.
- **A health warning**: some of the material in this text may bring up difficult thoughts, feelings and memories for the reader. I urge you to go gently and take good care of yourself on this journey.

2 My Story

So, who am I to write a book on trauma? As I have mentioned, I am a Clinical Psychologist by profession and have been studying and working with psychology and trauma for many years now. I began my professional journey in the mid-1990s when I embarked on a psychology degree at the University of East London as a mature student in my mid-20s. I went on to gain experience in the field of Clinical Psychology and pursue other life goals before finally completing my doctorate in Clinical Psychology in early 2007. I have worked with many hundreds of people in a therapeutic capacity and have been humbled many times by their stories of survival and perseverance in the face of great challenges. I have been proud to help so many of them find at least some relief from their pain and set them on a path to greater satisfaction and fulfilment in their lives. You might wonder what draws a person to work with other people's adversity. I am sure there are many reasons for many different people in my field, but for myself, I think a large part of the attraction lies in my own experiences of trauma and adversity. I think what drew me to psychology in the first place was a desire to understand my own rather complex trauma history and make meaning from it. The more I learnt, the more I wanted to bring that knowledge to others. As you will see, I had quite the journey to get to where I am today.

I grew up in a middle-class family in a middle-class village in the northwest of England. My family went to church, and my late father was a church warden for many years. My mother was a stay-at-home parent, and my father worked in an office. To the outside eye, it probably seemed like a typical family, with no obvious problems. We were neither especially rich nor poor and to all intents and purposes, we looked like an unexceptional family. Well, as we all know, appearances can be deceptive.

Behind closed doors, things were not as they should have been, and some of what I am about to discuss may bring up difficult feelings and may be triggering for some of you. My father was an angry man, and he took it out verbally and physically on his wife and children, more so on the boys. In his later years, he admitted that he was gay. Back in the 1960s, when my parents married, homosexuality was illegal in the UK and deeply stigmatised. Many gay men of that era hid their sexuality as much from themselves as from their families and wider society. Many of these men, including my father, married and brought up families as that was the only way to be deemed respectable. There has been very little open discussion in my family about these issues. My father never really spoke to me about anything, and certainly nothing as deeply personal as this. What I do know though is that this may have been one of the reasons that he was so angry and unreasonable with his wife (my mother), and his children.

I was always very afraid of my father and never really understood this fully. I recalled seeing him verbally and physically abusing my younger foster brothers on a regular basis and assumed that this, plus his generally angry behaviour and unpredictable moods, was the root of my fear. He was always very critical of everyone and especially seemed to take pleasure in misogynistic comments towards any female, including me. This made me want to try my best to please him and not invite his criticism, but at the same time I did not share his view of how women should behave and what they should aspire to. I was set up to fail here because the harder I tried to please him, the more I think I offended him. As a teenager I naturally became more rebellious and gave up trying to please him, it seemed to be a lost cause anyway.

In my early 40s, I began training in a trauma-focused therapy called Eye Movement Desensitisation and Reprocessing Therapy (EMDR). In one of the practicum sessions where we tested out our learning on each other, I was recalling and processing an innocuous minor trauma memory from school, when my mind took a leap back to a time when I was aged about six or seven when my father had yelled at me for using the bathroom when he wanted to use it and called me 'a stupid girl' among other things. That was a memory I had always been aware of and was moderately upset by, and I agreed to carry on with the processing in the hope of resolving that memory. Then my mind took another leap, to an unknown, dark place. I felt very small indeed, maybe about 18 months – 2 years old – playing in a bedroom with my, probably 3–4-year-old, older brother, making a blanket den to play in between the twin beds. Whilst processing, in the training session, I felt a sudden overwhelming sense of fear and then felt a sharp stinging pain on the side of my head and face and a falling sensation. With my adult eyes on the situation during the processing, I could see that my father had come into the room and told us off for playing when we should have been in bed, whilst nearly knocking toddler-me into the middle of next week with a flat handed blow across the side of my head. I felt immense anger and hurt, both physical and emotional, and it took quite some time for this to settle in the training session. To this day, I am a huge advocate of EMDR therapy largely because of my experience of both recalling and resolving such a traumatic event in the course of a single afternoon training workshop. EMDR can often resolve things like this very rapidly, and I was soon feeling a sense of relief and newfound comprehension. Later that month I had to visit my parents, something I always dreaded and avoided. I was really shocked to notice how much less anxious I felt in his presence and how I was able to breathe normally. Previously I would have been very, very tense, nervously holding my breath when near him. This explained to me why I had always been so scared of him even though I had not, until that moment in the EMDR training workshop, recalled him ever having hit me and had had no prior inkling of that specific event. For the doubters among you, I have fact-checked that event with significant others, and it has been confirmed that this event happened.

There were many instances of verbal and emotional abuse towards me, his dislike of females generally, and me in particular, was palpable. I was told I was worthless, just a girl, a useless girl, a stupid girl and so on, more times than enough. When you hear those things often enough part of you begins to believe them even whilst another part may know that it is not true. This destroyed my self-confidence and made me an easy target for the bullies during secondary school.

Trauma experts talk about traumatic stress being what happens when overwhelming events occur in the absence of an attuned other. A parent who can support you through adverse events and ease your distress can make all the difference to how severely trauma takes hold of you. I never felt adequately protected or supported, and I felt terribly alone with all this as a young person. I threw myself into my studies as a way of distracting myself from my feelings and to gain a sense of achievement. Feeling inadequate, worthless and stupid for being female drove me to want to prove something to … to whom? Myself? My father? I am not really sure what I wanted to prove, or to whom, but I do know that being a 'swot' did not make me popular with my peers at school! Nevertheless, it did give me a good educational foundation to deal with what came next.

As a lost and confused teenager, my main mission in life was to get away to college or university, escape from home and reinvent myself. I had been working part-time in a local hotel throughout my A-levels. My school and my father were pressuring me to do Oxbridge entrance exams to study modern languages or economics. However, I very much doubt that either 'Ox' or 'Bridge' would have been very impressed by my D in Economics A Level! I had other ideas anyway and in a rather pathetic attempt at a teenage rebellion, I opted instead to do a Catering Management Diploma at a Polytechnic college in Yorkshire. The first year was going fine, and I was really enjoying the freedom of being away from home. I quickly realised this was not where I belonged academically, but I did not really care at the time, I was making new friends and felt free of the turmoil of my earlier home life. Then for the summer term of 1986, I was sent off to do a work placement at a hotel in the Lake District where I was to be used as free student labour throughout the summer tourist season.

About a month into my placement, I contracted bacterial meningitis out of the blue, which came with side orders of sepsis and total organ failure. This resulted in the amputation of both legs above the knee due to gangrene caused by the disease. I spent about five weeks in intensive care, at least two weeks of which I was in an induced coma, and then I was in hospital for a further six to seven months gradually being put back together, and rehabilitated. I was left with significant scarring and physical disability. I have used a wheelchair ever since. Needless to say, this whole episode was extremely traumatic, and I was left with the very complicated task of processing what had happened, grieving the losses involved and reinventing myself as a disabled young woman in 1980s Britain.

When I was ready for discharge from the hospital, everyone assumed I would go home to my parents. I was not even asked and did not know that I had a choice. I was 19, newly disabled, and once again totally lost. I did go back to them, as I did not appear to have any choice at the time. Social services went in and tried to do some adaptations to the house to make it more accessible for me to return home to, which my father angrily resisted and obstructed. Once I was home, he then set about a campaign of making things as difficult as he could for me. I was using a wheelchair, and he would place obstacles in my way. He would move everyday items out of my reach so that I could not simply make myself a drink or do anything independently. If I transferred onto the sofa, he would take my wheelchair out of the room, in what I can only assume now was some sort of power-play. When I applied for Mobility Allowance, as it was then called, my father told me he was going to use it to lease a vehicle on the Motability Scheme. I very quickly put him straight and firmly told him it was *my* allowance, and *I* would be taking out the lease, for *my* car. Despite his abusive behaviour at this point, he would complain bitterly to anyone who would listen about the burden of care he had taken on in having me back home. I felt trapped and vulnerable. I also felt determined not to let this be the end of my story. Meningitis had failed to kill me, and I was not going to let my father destroy whatever life I was left with. I'm tempted to say 'what doesn't kill you makes you stronger' here, but I think that's another myth about trauma. In my case what didn't kill me left me disabled, angry and traumatised.

Within weeks I had phoned the local council housing office and had been placed on the waiting list for an accessible flat. I sorted out my disability benefit entitlements and was able, within months of being discharged from hospital, to lease a suitable car on the Motability Scheme. Motability is a UK-wide charitable scheme that enables disabled people to use their government benefits to lease vehicles at favourable rates. Luckily, I already had my driving license, and all I needed was a few additional driving lessons to familiarise myself with driving on hand controls. My newfound mobility allowed me to join a disabled persons' swimming club and a wheelchair basketball club. Sport and physical activity seemed to give me a renewed sense of being capable of something, a sense of well-being and a social support network full of role models for how to be a disabled person back in 1980s Britain. I went from complete novice to GB Women's Wheelchair Basketball team in about two seasons. I had a ten-year career with the GB Women's team, including representing Team GB at the Atlanta Paralympics in 1996, and alongside that, I played for various teams in the national league before taking a break to focus on other life goals. By the late 1990s, I had completed a degree in psychology at the University of East London and married my husband.

That last paragraph makes it sound like an easy process once I had the groundwork in place. In reality though, significant levels of anxiety and a lack of self-confidence plagued me throughout those years. The sense of not being worthwhile, or good enough, instilled in me by my father was never far from my mind. As an international athlete, I questioned my place on the team constantly, feeling that someone had made a mistake and I would be found out soon for the imposter I was. In my studies I worked exceptionally hard for fear of failing, when all along I was on course for a first-class honours degree. This imposter syndrome prevented me from publishing research that was worthy of publication and made me reluctant to apply for jobs that would further my desire to study Clinical Psychology. Part of me knew that I was more than able and that I had important things to say to the world, but another part of me would always question, 'But are you really worth it?', 'Are you good enough?', 'Do you deserve success?'

Around 1998/1999, my life moved away from basketball for a time, but I kept swimming for fitness and leisure as I began my career in psychology, moved back up north to Yorkshire with my husband and had my daughter. My daughter was born disabled, probably due to a severe kidney infection I had whilst pregnant. When she was about eight, we met up with some old friends from my wheelchair basketball days, and they encouraged us to go along to a training session. We were both immediately hooked and for me, it was as if I had never been away.

I qualified as a Clinical Psychologist in 2007 and began working with adults with trauma-related difficulties in the NHS, where I worked for many years. Since 2016 I have worked solely in private practice, offering treatment for trauma, as well as offering training and supervision to professionals working with trauma. My daughter is now an adult and still loves wheelchair basketball, playing in the team I now coach. I continue to swim, both at the gym and in open water.

I am incredibly grateful for the life I have now. I am happy to be ageing as I see growing old to be a privilege I very nearly missed out on. It was far from plain sailing to reach the point I am at now. There were many very difficult times dealing with low mood and anxiety, and a crippling lack of self-confidence at times. All of which is very typical for people living with the aftermath of trauma. Throughout this book, I hope to be able to share some of the things that have helped me to recover and cope with the extreme experiences I have lived through.

I would emphasise though that I do not have the perfect recipe for recovery. I experienced some severe bumps in the road getting to where I am now, and my solutions may not be right for you. Not everyone can take refuge in sport and exercise in the way I sometimes have. Not everyone has the academic skill or staying power to become a Clinical Psychologist. In fact, on reflection, some of my 'solutions' may even be seen as problematic in their own way. Striving so hard to achieve a very elusive career goal such as Clinical Psychology could be argued to be a symptom of the trauma I experienced growing up. What I mean by this is that growing up with so much criticism and emotional abuse meant that I had developed very low self-worth and was left with a feeling of needing to prove myself. I used my academic skills to strive to reach this seemingly insurmountable goal. Had I not experienced so much trauma growing up, I may have taken a different route entirely, with far less striving and more reasonable expectations of myself.

Nonetheless, I hope that the combined wisdom of my years of coping with trauma and treating others who are coping with trauma will be helpful to the reader.

Chapter Summary

- The author is a Clinical Psychologist with lived experience of trauma specialising in working in the field of trauma.
- The author had a very difficult childhood, followed by a severe and disabling illness at 19 years of age and has been a full-time wheelchair user since then.
- The author found refuge and community initially through sports and study.
- The author has had many struggles along the way, and what may seem at first glance to be a story of triumph over adversity is really not quite as simple as that.
- As the author of this book, I do not have all the answers, and I recognise that my answers may not work for everyone. Nonetheless, I have learnt from every person I have ever worked with and will be drawing on their wisdom too to help the reader find ways of coping with trauma.

3 Types of Trauma

What Does Trauma Really Mean?

As discussed in Chapter 1, trauma is a catch-all term for many different experiences. Colloquially, it can be used to describe everything from a lost wallet to the devastation of an earthquake. Teenagers, for example, are typically very dramatic in their descriptions of events and will describe the slightest mishap as a 'Trauma', a lost mobile phone, an outbreak of acne, a row with a partner, a fall out with a best friend, all feels very dramatic to the typical young person. As we get older, we learn to regulate our emotions better, and things seem less dramatic. Alternatively, trauma care is a significant area of physical medicine, referring to the physical treatment of broken bones, damaged limbs, brains and other organs following the impact of serious accidents. There is considerable overlap between physical health and psychological health here. For example, a traumatic brain injury may require both medical and psychological input in terms of assessment and treatment in order to achieve the best outcomes for the person affected. Similarly, the traumatic loss of a limb will require both surgical and medical intervention and will more than likely present psychological challenges to the person as they adjust to the loss and disability.

In psychology, we are interested in the emotional and behavioural aspects of a person's adjustment and recovery after something bad has happened, and this does not need to involve a major physical injury. Psychologists tend to think of trauma in bio–psycho–social terms, bio-meaning the biological, medical aspects; psycho- meaning the psychological, emotional and behavioural aspects; and the social referring to the person's wider environment of family, housing, access to amenities and activities and so on.

Within psychology, we may refer to T-traumas (big-T traumas) and t-traumas (little-t traumas). A T-trauma would present a very real threat to life and limb, a severe road or rail accident, a tsunami, a terrorist attack, active combat, humanitarian crisis or a bout of bacterial meningitis such as I experienced in my teens. Whereas a t-trauma would not in itself be life-threatening; it may be a one-off slap from a parent, a fight with peers in the playground, a minor road accident or a critical comment from a partner. In isolation, a t-trauma will be an upsetting experience that has little to no significant lasting impact. However, an unrelenting series of t-traumas can create a build-up of disturbance in a person's system that may have just the same effect as a single T-trauma.

Simple Trauma and Complex Trauma

Another distinction we make in psychology is between simple trauma and complex trauma. As this book is aimed at helping people cope with the effects of trauma, I am not going to labour the specifics of the diagnostic criteria for different types of trauma. In essence, simple trauma is likely to be a single incident traumatic event in adulthood, whereas complex trauma is exposure to either very extreme, prolonged traumatic events, or a series of very severe events particularly in childhood, while the person's sense of self is still developing, and these types of experiences have specific types of impact on a person. Post-traumatic stress disorder (PTSD) is a possible outcome of a simple traumatic event, whereas complex-PTSD is a likely outcome of complex trauma. To add to the confusion, the different diagnostic manuals (The American Psychiatric Association's DSM-5TR and the World Health Organisation's ICD-11) do not even recognise exactly the same diagnoses, and the criteria are slightly different in each and change with each revision of the manuals! Because of the complexity, I tend to use the concepts of trauma, complex trauma and post-traumatic stress very loosely in my general practice, and only really consider the strict diagnostic frameworks when I am requested to complete a legal report.

To give a little more context, a major incident such as a serious road or rail crash would be considered a T-trauma and, in isolation, may lead to a case of simple PTSD. As I outlined in Chapter 1, the person may experience many of the following symptoms:

- **Intrusions** – unwanted thoughts, images and body sensations both when asleep and awake including flashbacks and nightmares;
- **Avoidance** – trying not to think about the event, using substances and distraction to blot it out, or avoiding external reminders such as certain people, places or situations; one example might be to take a different route to work to avoid the accident site, even when the alternative route takes double the time;
- **Mood Difficulties** – negative self-beliefs ('It's my fault', 'I failed', 'I deserved it'), low mood and strong emotions such as fear, horror, anger, guilt and shame;
- **Hyperarousal Symptoms** – irritability, angry outbursts, hypervigilance, panic, restlessness and poor sleep.

These symptoms can be very disabling and can lead to the loss of employment, the breakdown of relationships and even suicide. In reality, even with an event such as a major road or rail crash, research suggests that only about a quarter to a third of survivors go on to develop diagnosable PTSD so it is far from a foregone conclusion that a serious event will lead to PTSD. Current UK National Institute for Clinical Excellence (NICE) Guidelines give the figures as follows:

> *Post-traumatic stress disorder (PTSD) develops after a stressful event or situation of an exceptionally threatening or catastrophic nature. It is a disorder that can affect people of any age. Around 25–30% of people experiencing a traumatic event go on to develop PTSD.*
>
> (NICE Guideline, 2018)

For some people, there will be a series of unfortunate events, all with the potential to cause simple PTSD, and these appear to act cumulatively so that a person may manage quite well after one, two or even three major events, but then the fourth event, perhaps even quite a minor event comparatively, may tip them over into experiencing the full array of PTSD symptoms. It would be impossible to say with any certainty which event really caused the PTSD or how much each event contributed to it, as it is the combination of factors that has led to the development of PTSD. It can be extremely difficult when assessing people who are making personal injury compensation claims as their Solicitors always want to know specifically which event caused the symptoms and what percentage of the symptoms are caused by events x, y and z. Trauma really is not that black and white, and the impact is far more nuanced than the legal profession would like us to say. The reality is that trauma acts cumulatively on the person, and the more trauma they have experienced, the more severe the outcome is likely to be when another traumatic event occurs. This phenomenon is reflected in the saying 'It was the last straw that broke the camel's back'.

Complex PTSD (c-PTSD) requires more than just a few simple traumatic events. It is most often diagnosed where there has been a significant amount of trauma during childhood or when a single event was so extreme and prolonged with no means of escape or relief that the person may have wished for death to escape it. Examples would include situations of captivity and torture, being trafficked for sexual abuse or being neglected and/or abused for a substantial period during childhood. When humans experience these more extreme forms of traumatic events, there are certain survival strategies that kick in that can make recovery more difficult. These will be described more fully in the next chapter.

Attachment Trauma

One specific type of complex trauma we come across clinically is the trauma caused by poor relationships in infancy and childhood, often referred to as attachment trauma. As I mentioned in Chapter 1, humans are not very well-designed animals in terms of our physical attributes for survival. This is even more true of human infants. Human babies are born very prematurely compared to most other mammals, the theory being that our comparatively huge brains mean that our heads would be too big to travel down the birth canal if we were kept in the womb long enough to develop our bodies more fully. Most mammalian babies are born ready to get to their feet and be able to find a food source or escape a predator quite soon after their birth. Human babies, on the other hand, are completely helpless for many months and cannot take care of themselves adequately for many years.

In the mid-twentieth century, John Bowlby, a Psychiatrist in London, began studying human attachment. He found that human infants, like all mammals, have an instinctive drive to attach to their caregivers and that the infant's well-being is severely and adversely affected by a poorer quality of attachment relationships (Bowlby, 1988). We know from Bowlby's early studies and the decades of subsequent research based on them that human infants experience neglect and abandonment as severely traumatic experiences. Part of the reasoning for this is that we are very vulnerable animals and rely very much on having a protective community around us to collaborate with for mutual survival. Abuse of all kinds can be traumatic, and this can be acts of commission or omission. By this I mean that a parent hitting a child (committing assault) will be traumatic to the child, but equally a parent neglecting a child (omitting to care) will also be traumatic to the child. Human infants have evolved an exceptionally strong drive to attach to their caregivers, and their wider family, for their sense of security and safety. If the caregivers are absent, or detached, the infant feels a threat to its very survival so will try to gain the attention of the caregiver or other family members using whatever skills are available to it. This might mean using aggression, crying or trying to appease the caregivers to attract attention and care. Even negative attention is preferable to no attention. Again, the child's logic is that if the caregivers are not paying attention, then I may as well have been left out for the wolves. Survival alone is impossible, so the child may as well give up and zone out in preparation for its inevitable demise. Once this zoning out becomes an established habit in the face of this kind of attachment trauma, it becomes a hard habit to break and tends to be an automatic reaction to any highly emotional state. We call this process of zoning out 'dissociation', and we will come back to it repeatedly throughout this book.

Intergenerational Trauma

There is a saying amongst trauma experts that 'hurt people can hurt people', meaning that those who have been hurt can go on to inflict hurt upon others, whether intentionally or not. I hasten to add that this is not a foregone conclusion, not all people who have been hurt go on to hurt others, if anything it would be a minority (Godsi, 1999). Nevertheless, if we have experienced poor attachments, neglect and abuse, it is possible that we will not have learnt how to do better when our own children come along, and we may unintentionally inflict harm upon them. We do sadly see examples of families where abuse and trauma are passed down like some sort of dreadful gift that just keeps on giving until the day someone decides to heal themselves and break the cycle. Gabor Maté, a Canadian Psychiatrist, originally from Hungary, and an expert on addictions, writes at length about the way a person who has experienced trauma in childhood may take refuge in drugs or alcohol to cope with their emotional pain (Maté, 2008). This abuse of substances then causes more pain and suffering within their present-day relationships and adversely impacts their ability to parent effectively. This knock-on effect can be passed on indefinitely, causing untold harm and suffering. We refer to this as the intergenerational transmission of trauma.

Trauma on a Global Scale

I was fortunate enough to hear Rolf Carrière speak at the EMDR UK conference in Liverpool in around 2016. Carrière is a retired Development Economist who has previously worked with the UN, the

World Bank in Asia, and for many years with Unicef in Bangladesh. He has discussed the importance of recognising and healing trauma on a global scale in his conference and TED talks. His TEDx talk at Groningen in 2013 (Carrière, 2013) covers much the same ground as the talk I saw him give. He describes how 'violence begets violence' and that being a victim of violence increases the risk of becoming a perpetrator of violence. He discusses the extent of political and criminal violence in the world, the extent of the refugee crisis, natural disasters, poverty and the scale of abuse against women. This was a hot topic in the 2010s, and the crises just seem to keep on escalating. As one war ends, another one begins. As climate change progresses, the world remains in denial, except for those directly affected by floods, droughts and famine. In his TEDx talk, Carrière stated some sobering UN statistics from 2011:

1.5 billion people were living with political and criminal violence
42 million refugees were internally displaced people
200 million people were affected by natural disasters
1.3 billion people were in absolute poverty
1 in 3 women were facing sexual, physical and other types of abuse

These figures will no doubt have increased since that time. Just to give one example, the UN Department of Economic and Social Affairs Statistics Division website states that 100 million people worldwide have been forcibly displaced in 2022, fleeing conflict, violence, human rights violations and persecution. As we are becoming increasingly aware, climate change is causing ever greater disturbance in many parts of the world, and people will inevitably be displaced and forced into extreme poverty as a result. Carrière is a strong advocate of EMDR as a scalable therapy that is effective and efficient and argues for much greater investment in bringing such treatment to those who need it. Other forms of therapy such as trauma-focused Cognitive Behavioural Therapy and Acceptance and Commitment Therapy have also demonstrated effectiveness in the treatment of trauma. However, sadly, I'm sure many readers are only too aware of how difficult it can be to access good-quality therapy for trauma.

Typical Trauma Responses

When faced with traumatic, life-threatening events, all mammals have a set of responses that have evolved to promote survival. Most people are familiar with the idea of the 'fight/flight' mechanism, whereby we feel fear or anger rising, our body becomes activated, our heart rate increases, our breathing speeds up and we feel primed for action, either to fight off the threat or to flee. During fight/flight, our mind becomes very focused on the immediate moment and how to get out of it in the best shape possible, we develop a sort of tunnel vision where all unnecessary processing or thinking is switched off. The survival advantage of flight/flight is that, assuming we are successful in winning the fight or fleeing safely, we either fight and overcome our enemies or we escape them. Either way, we live to fight another day and to bear offspring who will carry our genes forward. During fight/flight, our body releases hormones and brain chemicals to promote short-term strength, focus and pain relief. After the event, we can find that we have only a patchy recall of what happened or even total amnesia for the whole event, and we can find injuries we did not even realise we had sustained.

In addition to fight/flight, there are more trauma responses open to us. Where it seems impossible to survive or escape, we also have the freeze and flop responses. You may have seen wildlife documentaries where a small prey animal such as a baby antelope is being chased by a predator such as a cheetah. When the predator is gaining on the prey, often the prey will freeze or flop. A predator may not want to eat dead meat, as many prefer their meat fresh, and if the prey animal can convincingly play dead, the predator may just overlook it and reject it, so the baby antelope can escape to live another day. Alternatively, if the predator does catch the prey, part of the freeze or flop response is that the prey animal's system is flooded with pain-relieving brain chemicals, and the conscious, thinking mind is switched offline so it has little awareness of its final moments. We call this altered state of consciousness during trauma 'dissociation' and some degree of dissociation is common during most types of trauma. The more severe the event, the more likely it is that there will have been a significant amount of dissociation and as a result some people will have very little, if any, conscious recall of what happened.

In the case of attachment trauma, we also see the fawn response. Fawning is the attempt to placate the caregiver and to meet the caregiver's needs. The child's logic here is that by being a 'good kid' I may please my parents and thereby be rewarded with the care I need. This develops into a habit of people pleasing as the person grows up and can open them to further abusive and exploitative relationships. If fawning fails, the child may give up and adopt a freeze/flop response, becoming increasingly dissociated.

Chapter Summary

- Trauma means many different things to many people. It means something very different to a psychologist than to an orthopaedic doctor, and it means something very different to a typical teenager than to someone brought up in the care of a violent alcoholic parent.
- We refer to big-T traumas and little-t traumas as well as simple trauma and complex trauma.
- We have diagnostic categories, which have their uses, but generally, psychologists are more interested in what happened to someone, how distressed they are and how they can be helped with that, rather than which precise diagnostic box they can be squeezed into.
- Trauma can be an unwanted gift that keeps on giving! Sadly, some traumatised people will act out their pain by traumatising

others, keeping the cycle of trauma going generation upon generation.
- Trauma happens on an individual level, interpersonally, socially and globally, and there is a pressing need to reduce the burden of trauma on the world.

4 Impact of Trauma

In discussing the types of trauma we see clinically, I have already begun to describe some of the impacts we see. Trauma is not a black and white thing that you either have or you don't. As we have seen, a simple one-off event in adulthood can be traumatic, but set in the context of a healthy upbringing and a supportive social network, the impact may be relatively mild. The impact of an objectively lesser event in the context of a long history of neglect and poor relationships in the family background may be significantly more severe. While the formal diagnosis of post-traumatic stress disorder (PTSD) is an all or nothing outcome, you either meet the criteria or you don't, the experience of post-traumatic stress is very much on a spectrum from 'not at all affected' up to 'very severely disabling'. In addition to this, the way trauma affects us varies according to many factors such as our previous exposure to trauma, our personality prior to the event(s), the support we have after the event(s) and the sense we make of the event(s) to name but a few.

Further, the way our brain is wired from birth may impact our perception of, and reaction to, traumatic events. There is a group of conditions that I will categorise under the umbrella term of neurodivergence, which includes conditions such as autism, attention deficit hyperactivity disorder and learning disabilities which require special consideration when looking at the impact of trauma. I will discuss this in greater detail in Chapter 6.

ACE Studies (Adverse Childhood Experiences)

I have already mentioned that trauma has a cumulative impact on us and whereas a single event may be something we can recover quite easily from, a series of events can start to build up traumatic stress.

It's rather like an old-fashioned pressure cooker coming up to pressure and at some point, the pressure must be released, or the lid will blow off. The way the 'lid blows off' will vary for each of us because of our individual differences and experiences. Since the 1990s, there has been a steady stream of research coming out of the United States on the long-term impact of ACEs. This research began with Kaiser Permanente, a medical insurance company in the United States wanting to understand more about why people might have certain health problems in adulthood, including obesity. The aim of the original study was to identify preventable causes of ill health and intervene to improve health outcomes, with the aim of reducing health insurance pay outs. The ACEs studies began with a simple survey in an obesity clinic, asking whether people attending the clinic had experienced a certain set of events during childhood, including events like parental separation, parental violence, addictions and alcoholism within the family, physical or sexual abuse, bereavements and so on. The results were astonishing and have led to a great deal of further research on the impact of ACEs. Findings indicated that many physical health outcomes such as obesity correlate very highly with experience of early life trauma, with a clear exponential effect as the 'dose' of trauma increases (i.e. the more ACEs you have experienced, the worse your general health outcomes will be). See Figure 4.1, ACE Questionnaire.

In his now classic book *The Body Keeps the Score*, Bessel van der Kolk (van der Kolk, 2015) describes the ACE study and some of its shocking findings. The ACE study was initially carried out on mainly white, middle-class people in the United States with a good level of health insurance, so it is not even close to a representative sample of the US population. Nevertheless, one in ten respondents reported experiencing frequent verbal abuse in their childhood home, more than 25% reported experiencing frequent physical abuse in their childhood home, 28% of women and 16% of men reported some form of sexual assault during childhood and one in eight reported witnessing domestic violence against their mother (van der Kolk, 2015). The ACE Questionnaire consisted of ten items with one point per item scored.

Impact of Trauma

ACE Questionnaire

While you were growing up, during your first 18 years of life:

1. Did a parent or other adult in the household often or very often …
   Swear at you, insult you, put you down or humiliate you?
   or
   Act in a way that made you afraid that you might be physically hurt?
   Yes No   If yes enter 1 _____

2. Did a parent or other adult in the household often or very often …
   Push, grab, slap or throw something at you?
   or
   Ever hit you so hard that you had marks or were injured?
   Yes No   If yes enter 1 _____

3. Did an adult or person at least five years older than you ever …
   Touch or fondle you or have you touch their body in a sexual way?
   or
   Attempt or actually have oral, anal, or vaginal intercourse with you?
   Yes No   If yes enter 1 _____

4. Did you often or very often feel that …
   No one in your family loved you or thought you were important or special?
   or
   Your family didn't look out for each other, feel close to each other or support each other?
   Yes No   If yes enter 1 _____

5. Did you often or very often feel that …
   You didn't have enough to eat, had to wear dirty clothes and had no one to protect you?
   or
   Your parents were too drunk or high to take care of you or take you to the doctor if you needed it?
   Yes No   If yes enter 1 _____

6. Were your parents ever separated or divorced?
   Yes No   If yes enter 1 _____

7. Was your mother or stepmother:
   Often or very often pushed, grabbed, slapped or had something thrown at her?
   or
   Sometimes, often, or very often kicked, bitten, hit with a fist or hit with something hard?
   or
   Ever been repeatedly hit for at least a few minutes or threatened with a gun or knife?
   Yes No   If yes enter 1 _____

FIGURE 4.1 The ACE Questionnaire. Source: Adapted from Shapiro (1990; revised 2021).

> 8. Did you live with anyone who was a problem drinker or alcoholic or who used street drugs?
> Yes No   If yes enter 1 _____
> 9. Was a household member depressed or mentally ill, or did a household member attempt suicide?
> Yes No   If yes enter 1 _____
> 10. Did a household member go to prison?
> Yes No   If yes enter 1 _____
> Now add up your 'Yes' answers: _____ This is your ACE Score.

FIGURE 4.1 (Continued)

One in six of the respondents had an ACE score of four or higher. Given that this was a relatively privileged sample of the US population (i.e. mostly white people in good jobs with good health insurance cover), it is fair to assume that the scores would be considerably higher among populations experiencing the additional challenges of racism, poverty, disability or other forms of exclusion. What this clearly demonstrates is that traumatic life experiences in childhood are remarkably common, even in relatively privileged communities, which is precisely what Freud tried to tell us back in the 1890s.

The initial ACE study has been built upon by further research to explore the different outcomes that people experience when scoring highly for ACEs. The studies show strong correlations between raised ACE scores and poor academic achievement, behavioural problems, chronic depression, imprisonment, substance misuse, chronic ill health and early death. The logic of this can be seen in Figure 4.2 (the ACEs Pyramid). Being born to someone with an existing trauma history means that you will more than likely experience poorer social conditions and adverse experiences, which impact your brain development causing impairments in your social, emotional and cognitive development. Typically, this results in unhealthy behaviours such as poor eating patterns or substance misuse, which lead to disease and disability and ultimately reduced life expectancy.

Impact of Trauma

```
                    Death
         Early
         Death
      Disease,
     Disability, &
   Social Problems
      Adoption of
  Health Risk Behavior
    Social, Emotional,
   & Cognitive Impairment
   Disrupted Neurodevelopment
   Adverse Childhood Experiences
   Social Conditions / Local Context
 Generational Embodiment / Historical Trauma
                                              Conception
Mechanism by which Adverse Childhood Experiences
Influence Health and Well-being Throughout the Lifespan
```

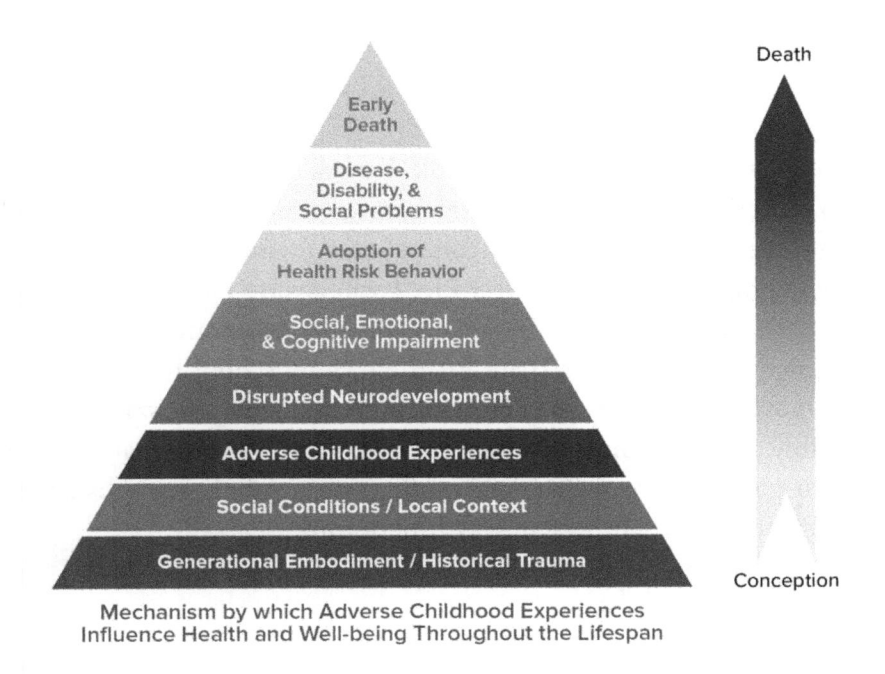

FIGURE 4.2 The ACE Pyramid. Source: Centre for Disease Control (CDC).

To illuminate this trajectory with an example, imagine an abused young woman brought up in the social care system, let's call her Jenny. Without guidance or support, Jenny gets pregnant at a young age and has a son, let's call him Jake. Jenny cannot afford to live in a safe, prosperous neighbourhood and is unable to secure well-paid work due to childcare demands and poor academic achievement resulting from having left school early to have Jake. Jake then faces poor social conditions and may experience abuse from Jenny's later partner(s) or the neighbourhood gangs. Jake is traumatised, and this disrupts his development, adversely impacting his schooling. Jake becomes disruptive at school as no one appears to notice how much he is struggling, all that is noticed is his poor behaviour, and this is treated with punishment and exclusion. Jake's bad behaviour escalates, and as he reaches his teens or possibly even sooner, he discovers drugs and alcohol, and in all likelihood the cycle will repeat with criminality, incarceration and poor health outcomes being very likely. Sadly, as discussed in

Chapter 3, trauma and abuse are unwanted gifts that keep on giving, and in trauma therapy circles this is known as the intergenerational transmission of trauma.

What I see clinically in the people I work with is that the different manifestations of distress can almost invariably be linked back to adverse experiences. When someone comes to me experiencing difficulty coping in their day-to-day life, I will always take some time to explore their background with them. I am curious about what life was like growing up, who was there for them, how school was and what difficult experiences they may have encountered along the way. Almost invariably there is some history of trauma and adversity and when we then go on to process the old trauma, we regularly see substantial improvements in their present-day functioning.

My ACEs Profile

Looking through the ACE Questionnaire above, I can confidently score myself with four, or maybe five, ACEs and this does not even consider the massive medical trauma I experienced at 19 years of age when I caught meningitis and lost my legs. From the ACE studies we know that there is a dose effect with trauma and that the more ACEs and traumas a person has experienced, the more likely they are to have adverse outcomes in life. However, this is not a foregone conclusion, and I think I am living proof that a tough childhood and a severe trauma do not necessarily have to mean a lifetime of low achievement, depression and poor health. There are many influencing factors, the most important of which is probably luck. Luck meant that I was white British, academically capable, living in the UK, with good education and healthcare opportunities. Although not wealthy, my family was averagely comfortable financially, so despite the discord within the home, there was a good quality house, in a good neighbourhood with good schools nearby. I wonder how different my post-trauma experiences might have been had I been brought up in a less privileged environment where I had to face poverty or racism in addition to my other difficulties.

As I explained in the previous chapter, Psychologists often talk about formulating people's difficulties using a 'Bio–Psycho–Social Model'. From this perspective, biologically I must have been pretty robust to have survived a near-fatal dose of meningitis, probably because I had always had good healthcare via the UK's National Health Service. I was generally well-fed and physically well taken care of from infancy; then I had the good fortune to have my illness recognised, diagnosed and treated rapidly and effectively. Psychologically, as a teenager, I was vulnerable and could easily have gone down the route of severe and escalating depression and anxiety. The home I grew up in was not happy, emotions were not welcomed or discussed at all, and there was an expectation that if something went wrong, you just had to 'get on with it'. Then socially, although my family life was always very challenging, I also had social advantages such as my intellect, education, healthcare and white privilege to get me through. So clearly the picture is not as simple as a certain score on the ACE Questionnaire determining a certain trajectory in life. Being human is a lot more complicated than that!

Intersectionality

In social psychology and sociology, there is the concept of intersectionality to capture the complexity of the human experience. Typically, humans think in very binary terms, people are black or white, able or disabled, rich or poor, clever or stupid, gay or straight. However, very little of human experience is as simple or binary as that (Barker & Iantaffi, 2019). Each person's experience will consist of many different characteristics which all intersect differently at various places along each spectrum. Where I may experience privilege due to some aspects of my make up, I may be oppressed due to others, or I may fall somewhere in-between. The point I am trying to emphasise here is that we are all far more than just the sum of our ACE scores, or any other questionnaire a psychologist may put in front of us. It is the sum of our experience in all its complexity that will determine how we are impacted by our experience of trauma.

Linking Past Trauma to Present Difficulty

The sort of problems people present with in my therapy clinic are many and varied, the most common being:

- anxiety and depression
- anger management
- disordered eating
- difficult relationship with alcohol or drugs
- self-image and self-esteem problems
- obsessive-compulsive behaviours
- relationship difficulties
- fears and phobias
- chronic fatigue and pain conditions, often with no obvious medical cause.

Additionally, because I specialise in treating trauma-related issues, many people seek me out and present to me specifically because they recognise that trauma plays a part in their current difficulty, and they already know they want to deal with that.

It is not always immediately obvious to the person seeking help how their past links to their current difficulty, but this usually becomes clearer as therapy progresses. When adverse events happen, we go into a survival mode, as discussed in the previous chapter. Our system shuts down any unnecessary processes to preserve every possible ounce of energy for the fight or flight. The human thinking brain normally uses a large amount of energy – pondering, daydreaming, working things out, planning and strategising. All of this activity would get in the way of effective fight/flight behaviour and would use up too much energy, so it quietens down and our more instinctive reptilian and mammalian brain processes take over to get us through the emergency as intact and alive as possible. The result of this is that our experience is not fully processed and is not filed away neatly during the traumatic event in a coherent and sensible way, rather, we are left with a fragmented jumble of information in the form of thoughts, feelings, body sensations and images, all just thrown in the back of our mind somewhere to be sorted through and filed away later when the immediate danger is over. In an ideal situation, sometime after the event the person can take some time to process what has happened, by thinking about it, talking about it with friends and family and dreaming about it during sleep. These processes should allow the fragmented bits of memory to be joined together rather like a jigsaw puzzle, any missing pieces retrieved and the memory filed away under the heading of 'bad things that have happened that I have processed and feel alright about', and the person can move on with minimal ongoing distress. Unfortunately, however, it doesn't always work out like that for the bigger traumatic events.

When something very bad happens, it overwhelms our ability to cope, we often don't want to think about it, we try to shut out memories and thoughts, we try to distract ourselves with busy activity or numb the thoughts and feelings with drugs or alcohol. We avoid talking about the event because to do so overwhelms us again, and the events can be highly distressing for our friends and family to hear so we try to protect them from it. Our mind may try to resolve things by dreaming about the event while we sleep, but the dreams become nightmares and wake us up in a hot sweat and a state of panic, unsure where we are and whether the awful thing is happening all over again. Thus, we are unable to complete the processing because we wake up before it is resolved and then we become too scared to sleep, and we will try anything to stay awake. This situation can rapidly escalate into full-blown PTSD. The more we avoid thinking about the event and talking about the event, the more it tries to intrude into our awareness, with intrusive thoughts and images, flashbacks, nightmares and emotional upset. In the same way that our body is designed to heal most injuries, our mind is also designed to heal itself. Our mind knows that it needs to relive the experience in some form to learn and heal from it and make meaning from what has happened. A part of our mind wants to try and process the memory and file it away, but at the same time another part wants to avoid going there, and this becomes a vicious cycle with greater avoidance leading to increased intrusions, making us try to avoid it all the more. At this point there is an escalating battle going on, and the traumatic event is rapidly becoming the only thing that person can think about. Judith Herman in her 1992 book *Trauma and Recovery* calls this the 'dialectic of trauma' meaning that the traumatised person swings between a sort of numbing out or denial, and reliving of the event(s).

Chapter Summary

- Trauma impacts us all very differently depending on our circumstances and the type of traumatic events we have experienced.
- Neurodivergent people (i.e. those with autism, ADHD, and learning disabilities) experience trauma differently than neurotypical people (i.e. those without those conditions).
- The ACE studies demonstrate how trauma can impact all areas of personal well-being such as physical and mental health, life expectancy, career and educational attainment and social status.
- My own experience shows that individual outcomes are mediated by a range of personal characteristics and how they intersect with each other.
- Clinically, people present with conditions such as anxiety, low mood, anger, disordered eating, addictions, obsessions and compulsions, relationship difficulties, fears and phobias and medically unexplained health problems, much of which can be traced back to unresolved traumatic experiences.
- Trauma overwhelms our ability to cope, and we try to shut out the experience, leading to the development of clusters of symptoms that will only fully resolve when we address the trauma.

5   Added Complexity

So far, I have described some of the more typical trauma presentations we see clinically. In cases where there has been more damaging early abuse and neglect, we tend to see a more complex picture in the people who present for help. These people still initially present with the standard problems of anxiety, low mood, disordered eating, substance misuse, obsessions, compulsions, fears and phobias, or chronic, unexplained ill health, but as we work together it becomes apparent that there are opposing forces within the person that make treatment more difficult. There are parts of the person that are somewhat disconnected from each other and appear to be acting independently and, at times, in conflict with each other. What seems to happen is that when children go through traumatic events, it is as though they leave a 'part' of themselves hidden away in their mind, holding on to the memory and the feelings associated with it, stuck at the age when it happened, frozen in time. In some cases, this may happen many times, and there may be many 'parts' of the self, hidden away to a greater or lesser extent in the mind, representing different events at different ages (Boon, Steele & van der Hart, 2011). To a degree this is completely normal, most of us will have a sense in our minds of our 'five-year-old self starting school', or our '11-year-old self moving up to high school' or our 'teenage self' discovering relationships or alcohol for the first time. The difference here is that there is some sense of coherence for most of us, a sense that the five-year-old self is just us at a younger age. For people who have experienced severe early trauma, there can be much more of a disconnect between the 'parts' and less of a sense that 'that is just me at that age'. In trauma therapy, we talk about these parts as being dissociated parts of the personality, separated off when the trauma occurred to protect the person growing up from the distress of the memory.

Ego/Self States and Internal Family Systems

This sort of fragmentation of the self has been described in different ways over the years by many different theorists. In 1997, Watkins and Watkins wrote about 'Ego State Therapy', where they used hypnosis to access the dissociated parts and bring them into dialogue with each other, bringing past traumatic events into consciousness in the process. In Cognitive Analytic Therapy (Ryle, 1995), part of the process of understanding the presenting problem is to map out the 'multiple self states' that take over the person and hijack their best intentions. In Internal Family Systems Therapy (Schwartz, 2001; Schwartz & Sweezy, 2020), it is understood that we are all made up of multiple parts and that trauma creates disruption in the smooth running of the 'internal family system' with some parts being exiled, some parts taking protective roles to hide traumatic memories from awareness and other parts leaping in with knee jerk reactions to deal with emergency situations (triggers). All these explanations are attempts to understand the complexity of people who have experienced terrible trauma.

For me, this complexity is best described by Janina Fisher in her book *Healing the Fragmented Selves of Trauma Survivors* (Fisher, 2017). She describes how the self becomes fractured, with parts holding onto traumatic memories and unbearable emotion of early life siloed off out of awareness, while a 'going about daily business' part of the self presents as normal a front to the world as possible. The difficulty is that these siloed off parts can become activated, or triggered, by new situations that are reminiscent of the original trauma, and the person gets a sense of being 'taken over' or losing control. An example of this is the apparently capable business executive, let's call him Dave, who becomes a quivering wreck when the boss calls him into the office. Dave feels like he is going to cry or wet himself and feels terrible fear and shame. What appears to be happening here is that a child part, possibly abused in the past by a domineering parent, is being activated by the sense of threat when an authority figure (i.e. the boss) calls him into the office. A particular child part of Dave then thinks he's going to be in trouble because that was always the case if his father summoned him. His child part cannot distinguish between 'dad then' and 'boss now' and cannot recognise that he is now a grown man who can look after himself. The work of therapy then is to enable Dave to process the trauma of the past so that his childhood part no longer needs to work so hard to protect his adult self. There are many ways to work on this in therapy, and even very severely fragmented minds can be treated with a patient and compassionate approach.

Dissociative Identity Disorder

At the most extreme end of the spectrum of trauma presentations, we see people whose personalities have fractured to such an extent that their dissociated parts are acting independently of each other, taking over control of everyday life. We call this kind of presentation Dissociative Identity Disorder (DID) (Boon, Steele & van der Hart, 2011). In cases of DID the fragmentation is more complete and there will be little to no awareness between the parts of each others' existence. This can lead to severe difficulties functioning in everyday life. DID has been a controversial diagnosis as many Psychiatrists and some Psychologists do not believe it exists. However, if you feel that this discussion really resonates with your experiences, you will likely find that self-help alone will not be sufficient to resolve your complex history of trauma. I would encourage you to find a suitably trained practitioner to give you some additional help. I could not write a book on coping with trauma without at least mentioning this important area, and I hope that some of the strategies I will put forward will be beneficial as you start your healing journey.

Trauma Isn't Binary

I have already alluded to trauma presentations being on a spectrum, rather than an all-or-nothing binary, and I think this is a helpful way to think of it. For some people, who have a reasonable, good enough family background, even quite a severe traumatic event might be easily processed, and the person may not go on to have many difficulties at all from it. At the other end of the spectrum, we have those people who have experienced a severely neglectful and abusive early life whose entire personality has been fractured into many dissociated parts and have little sense of a coherent identity. There are many ways that trauma can present in between these two extremes, and I would argue that at the heart of many, many mental health struggles that we see in clinical settings, there will be some history of trauma that underpins much of the difficulty we see. Which, again, is what Freud tried to tell us back in the 1890s.

Richard Schwartz who writes about Internal Family Systems (IFS) Therapy takes the view that we are all a multiplicity of parts and that getting to know our inner world better is healing for all of us. He argues that we all have hidden parts and that depending on the degree of trauma we have experienced our inner world may be anything from relatively straightforward all the way through to extremely complex and fragmented.

IFS from the Inside

In writing about these issues, I was reminded that I wanted to explore this aspect of my own mind in more depth and embarked on a course of IFS therapy with a colleague. I am very aware of my privilege in being able to access this and pay for it without having to wait months or years on an NHS waiting list and being able to choose the style of therapy I want, to address the issues as I see them. One of the reasons I am writing this book is to impart some of these lessons to people who are not able to access therapy so that they can learn to cope better with their trauma.

As I am writing this chapter, I am only a few sessions into that course of therapy, but already there have been many revelations and tears. I have become aware of a very busy part of myself that can never rest and is always looking for the next task to take on. That part is

Added Complexity

trying to prove herself to be good enough, or even more than good enough, to overcome the doubts placed in her mind by her hyper-critical, misogynistic, emotionally abusive father. At the same time, there is a very tired part of myself that craves sofas and blankets and mindless TV. That part recognises that I have been running away from my childhood for decades now and am exhausted from my efforts to prove myself and achieve beyond all doubt. The struggle between these two parts leaves me quite conflicted at times. Busy-me wants to see 20 people a week for therapy and supervision, and help out facilitating on trainings, and run supervision groups, and write a book, and coach wheelchair basketball, and look after my daughter, and run the house, and ..., and ..., and ...! Whilst tired me just wants a nice glass of wine and a snooze on the sofa with a snuggly woollen blanket. These parts pull me in different directions so that when my busy part is active I can feel frustrated that I am not caring well for myself or my family, whilst when the tired part takes over I feel guilty for not getting things done. Sometimes it feels like I can't win with myself, I am sure there will be far more insights as I progress through this course of therapy.

Getting to know your inner world first requires skills in relaxation and an openness to experiencing emotions and difficult memories. It is not something to launch into unsupported without taking time to prepare yourself and test the waters gently. Before I introduce you to an exercise where you can begin to connect with your inner world, I am going to introduce you to some basic relaxation techniques. These will need to be practiced, and your tolerance for them will need to be built up gradually before you delve into any deeper work on yourself. Most relaxation techniques involve paying attention to our breathing and to our body sensations. There are many such exercises available to download on the internet, and it may help you to find guided relaxation exercises that you can listen to. I have listed some useful resources in Chapter 16 to help with this. For most of us, we find that concentrating on our breathing naturally causes our bodies to slow down and relax. When we are tense, we tend to shallow breathe, just taking in air to the top of our lungs and not fully exhaling the air from the bottom of our lungs. Making the effort to breathe all the way down to our abdomen and fully exhale for a few minutes can be deeply relaxing. Try it now.

1. Settle into a comfortable, upright position on a chair or cushion. You may prefer to close your eyes.
2. Notice the feeling of your breath as it enters your nose.
3. Follow the breath as it travels down the back of your throat, into your chest and feel the muscles of your chest wall expand as you draw the air in deeper.
4. Notice your abdomen expand as the air fills your chest cavity.
5. Feel the briefest of pauses as your breath turns around and begins to leave the body.
6. Follow the breath back up out of the chest and let it out slowly through the mouth.
7. Repeat, following each breath, slowly and gently, not forcing anything.
8. You may only manage two to three breaths to begin with before you lose concentration, or feel uncomfortable, but with practice this should increase until you can concentrate on your breathing for several minutes.

Another way of learning to relax is to focus on your body. We often hold tension in our body and this can cause chronic pain if we ignore it and do not pay attention to it. Many trauma survivors especially carry large amounts of tension in their bodies, without realising it, as a result of being caught in a fight/flight response to multiple daily triggers. Learning to relax can feel scary at first as there is the belief that if you let your guard down for a moment, something awful will happen. Gradual exposure to relaxation is needed to build the skill over time. Progressive muscle relaxation is a simple way of beginning to tune into your body and notice where the tension is held and let it go. Try it now.

1. Find a comfortable place either sitting or lying on a chair or bed, or even on the floor on a yoga mat.

2. You may wish to close your eyes, but this is not essential.
3. Take a few relaxing breaths as described above as you settle into position.
4. Bring your attention to the muscles of your head and face, tighten those muscles for two to three seconds, scrunching your eyes and face as you do so and then let the tightness go as you breathe out slowly.
5. Move your awareness to the muscles of your neck and shoulders, tighten those muscles for two to three seconds and then let the tightness go on the out breath.
6. Move your attention to the muscles of your arms and hands, tighten the muscles for a couple of seconds and then let the tightness go as you breath out.
7. Bring your attention to the muscles of your chest and upper back, tighten them and let them go as you breath out.
8. Notice the muscles of your stomach and lower back, tighten and let go, just as before.
9. Notice the muscles of your pelvic area and bottom, tighten and let go, just as before.
10. Pay attention to the muscles of your legs and feet, tighten them and let them go as you breathe out.
11. Just take a few moments to rest in the relaxed state you find yourself in, noticing how your body has softened and let go of tension.

When you have practiced mindful breathing and progressive muscle relaxation and feel able to spend time in a calm relaxed state without feeling agitated or distressed, then you can move on to exploring your inner world in more detail.

Fraser's Table Exercise

Appreciating that not everyone can simply book in with a private therapist and start work on their fragmented parts, I am going to introduce an exercise here that can be done in the comfort of your own home. Most people can safely dabble with this exercise, but if you have a severe trauma history, engage in self-harm or other risky behaviour, or have a sense that you dissociate to a significant degree, then please seek professional help before trying this exercise.

In 1991, George A Fraser MD wrote a paper outlining a technique for working with this kind of multiplicity (Fraser, 1991). This has since become known as Fraser's Table Technique, and many variations on the theme have been developed since the 1990s. The aim of such techniques is to enable more joined up, flexible working of the person's inner system to develop harmony between parts, not to eliminate or necessarily integrate their parts.

The process usually starts with some explanation and then some coaching and practice in using relaxation techniques, as described above. Next the therapist encourages the person, in their relaxed state, to imagine a room with a large oval table and a number of chairs placed around it. The person is encouraged to imagine themselves in the room, taking a seat at the table and then to invite the parts of themselves of which they are aware to join them and take the remaining seats. For myself in this imagery, I imagine my toddler self, my 6–7-year old self, a 12–13-year old me, a 14–15-year old me and a version of me when I was in the hospital at 19 years old, then perhaps a few more versions of me from adulthood, and my current self. Other versions of me might join the group at a later stage, but off the top of my head these are the important parts of me that carry important parts of my story. They are all relatively well joined up these days, but that was not always the case for me. Before I trained in EMDR and had my profound experience during the training workshop described in Chapter 2, I would not have even thought of a toddler-me as being important and would not have invited her into the room. It is important to note that the parts may vary not just in age, but in gender, race and other aspects of identity. As an example, a person of mixed heritage may have a white western part that conforms to white western norms, whilst also having parts representing other parts of their heritage, conforming to different cultural norms. If these parts can get to know each other and enter into healthy dialogue, then any conflict can be resolved within the system, and the person can develop a more coherent sense of identity.

For people without a complex trauma history, this process can be a fun, revealing insight into their inner world and can help open up dialogue between, for example, the part that wants to lose weight and the part that raids the fridge at all hours of the night. The parts can learn to pass a microphone around the imagined table and take turns to speak, to tell their story, address their fears and hopes and resolve their differences (inner conflicts). In the process of talking to parts of the self, inevitably people begin to recall old memories. Our minds work by association, one thought triggers another thought, which triggers another thought and so on. We cannot pay attention to all our memories at once, but when we start thinking about one memory, we then remember another and another. This gradual unfolding, if done with caution and patience, can help someone to understand their inner conflicts and unconscious processes and begin to resolve them.

Fraser's paper goes on to describe some of the therapeutic interventions a therapist can make to enable greater understanding and coherence between parts. He describes a process of encouraging the parts to fuse together which we do not encourage so strongly nowadays, as we aim more towards cooperation and coherence between parts rather than fusion of parts. Nowadays, we recognise that we are all somewhat split and as long as our parts can work together for the common good, that is all that is needed. Janina Fisher, who also writes extensively about working with dissociated parts certainly doesn't recommend any intention to fuse or join parts, beyond fostering coherence and cooperation (Fisher, 2017).

Complexity and Risk

Fisher (2017) tells us that the therapy and mental health world has, until recently, been generally unreceptive to the idea that personalities and identities can be fragmented, and so therapists typically were not trained to recognise this aspect of their client's presentation, and many are not equipped to work effectively with these sorts of presentations. Often the fragmentation leads to severe conflicts within the person, and this can present as suicidal behaviour, self-harm, disordered eating and addictions, so these people are often the hardest to help and cause the most concern within medical and mental health services. The conflicted behaviour of a severely traumatised and fragmented individual often attracts punitive and restrictive treatment from services, which ultimately only adds to the burden of trauma that individual is carrying. Not surprisingly these people struggle to manage in education or the workplace and so have fewer resources to cope with the challenges of adult life. Sadly, in the UK since 2010, over successive governments, we have seen punitive cuts to all forms of welfare and mental health support, meaning that these people are being further traumatised by an unforgiving social environment, where there is a lack of compassion or support emanating from the heart of government throughout society.

Gabor Maté similarly describes his work with addicts in downtown Vancouver, Canada (Maté, 2008). Parts of his clients want a better life for themselves, but their wounded child parts seek oblivion and pain relief through the excessive use of drugs and alcohol. Their lifestyles then invite risk in the form of violence, disease, rejection and abandonment. They waver between trying to abstain and recover and needing the pain relief of their chosen substance to blot out the emotional and physical pain of their existence. Their lifestyles of addiction, periods of abstinence and constant relapse mean they are considered hard to help and attract further trauma from health services who become exasperated with their inability to stay sober or clean for more than a week or two at a time. Maté explains that practically every one of the people he works with describes a childhood full of some degree of neglect, violence and/or sexual abuse. The sad truth is that early trauma lies at the heart of so many of these tragic stories.

Chapter Summary

- Early trauma leads to fragmentation of the self, with parts of the self holding on to images, memories, thoughts and feelings of the past, often acting in conflict with other parts of the same self.
- Many theorists have described fragmentation in terms of ego states, multiple self states, IFS or simply parts.
- Relaxation skills are a first step to being able to connect with your inner world.
- Fraser's Table Exercise is a way to start connecting with your inner parts and opening up dialogue between your parts to resolve conflicts and generate greater harmony within.
- With added complexity of trauma comes added risk. People with the severest trauma histories will have parts that want to destroy the self, or at least shut out all reality. This means self-harm, suicidal acts and drug and alcohol misuse are common in this population, making them the hardest people to help, but also the ones who need the help the most.

6 Trauma and the Brain

Neurobiology of Trauma

The brain is a very complex structure, and for most of history, until the end of the twentieth and beginning of the twenty-first century, we have had very little knowledge of how it works. To be brutally honest, we still don't understand much, but our knowledge is growing all the time and has grown exponentially since the 1990s. As a Clinical Psychologist specialising in the treatment of trauma, I need to have a passing acquaintance with developments in neurobiology and how these can inform our understanding of trauma, and its treatment. I hope to convey in this chapter some of the key insights we have gained in the field of trauma therapy from the field of neurobiology. My aim here is to give an overview for the majority of readers and point the more curious reader towards other sources of literature where they may begin a deeper dive into this fascinating but complex science should they so desire.

Early History

Earlier scientists were able to infer some brain functions from the symptoms reported after brain injury. One famous example of this is the case of Phineas Gage, a railway construction worker in mid-nineteenth century America, who was injured when a metal rod was shot through his head in a horrific workplace accident. Remarkably he survived, and his story has long been a standard entry in most introductory psychology textbooks (e.g. Gross, 1992). His doctors at the time reported changes to his personality, including poor impulse control and loss of manners and etiquette. However, they also reported little damage to his other functions such as movement and intellect. Such stories have helped neuroscientists identify which parts of the brain control which functions, long before brain imaging technology was developed. Similarly, cases of speech impairment or memory loss following specific illnesses, injuries or surgery have helped scientists map out the functions of different brain areas. This endeavour was always rather rough and ready and relied on accidents or illnesses occurring to unfortunate people for learning to progress. In addition, the specifics of the injury could not be fully known until an autopsy of the injured brain was conducted, sometimes decades after the original injury.

The late, great British neurologist Professor Oliver Sacks wrote numerous fascinating texts on case studies in neuropsychology including Awakenings (Sacks, 1990), The Man Who Mistook His Wife for a Hat (Sacks 1985), Seeing Voices: A Journey into the World of the Deaf (Sacks, 1989), An Anthropologist on Mars (Sacks, 1995), to name but a few. Some of his works have formed the basis of movies and television documentaries. His career began with his medical degree from Queen's College, Oxford, in 1958, and his case studies are drawn from his subsequent clinical work in neurology in San Francisco and New York. His career spanned the decades just prior to the explosion of technological ways of seeing inside the living brain. They are nonetheless intriguing and offer the reader an accessible, often highly entertaining route into understanding some of the things that can go awry with the human brain.

Recent Technological Advances

The latter decades of the twentieth century saw tremendous advances in the ability of medics and neuroscientists to look inside our brains whilst we are alive and awake without the need for death or any injury to occur. Since the late twentieth and early twenty-first centuries, brain imaging studies have begun to show key structures and pathways in the brain which help us deal with emergencies and traumatic events. This is a rapidly developing and fascinating field of study which stands at the intersection between neuroscience and psychology. Advances in neuroscience have allowed psychologists to learn what happens in the brain when humans are faced with disturbing situations, traumatic imagery or reminders of traumatic events (van der Kolk, 2013). Clearly it would be unethical to severely traumatise research participants just to see what happens, and there are strict safeguards in place these days to protect research participants from harm. Nonetheless, researchers do use memories of mild to moderate trauma, or imagery from movies and news reports to elicit emotional reactions in research participants. These reactions can be tracked in the brain in real time using technology such as functional Magnetic Resonance Imaging (fMRI) to see which pathways and brain regions light up under different experimental conditions.

Dr Bessel van der Kolk, a psychiatrist in Boston, Massachusetts, was one of the first to use fMRI to map what happens when people recall traumatic events back in the mid-1990s. He discovered that during recall the visual cortex and emotional centres of the limbic system lit up noticeably, whilst the brain's speech centre was significantly less activated. In fact, the activity was largely located in the right brain with the left brain largely deactivated. What this tells us is that during traumatic recall, e.g. flashbacks, our ability to put the experience into words and apply logic is impaired, and we are taken over by emotional, visceral and visual stimuli. A control condition, where participants recalled a neutral or pleasant event, showed very different activation in the brain, with both sides activated in a more balanced way. Van der Kolk outlines this study in his 2015 book *The Body Keeps the Score*.

The Triune Brain

Based on our understanding so far in this rapidly evolving field, psychologists are now able to plot how different parts of the brain fire off or go quiet under different conditions. For convenience, psychologists think of the brain in terms of three main parts, assumed to have evolved at different stages in our evolutionary history. This conceptualisation dates back to the 1960s when neuroscientist Dr Paul MacLean, at Yale University School of Medicine, mapped out his model of the Triune Brain (for an overview see MacLean, 1990). MacLean's model has been criticised as an oversimplification of the workings of a very complex organ, and his idea that the different parts of the brain evolved at different times has been strongly challenged. However, the triune brain model is still widely used to make the complexity of neuroscience more accessible to those outside of the field of study. No model of brain function is ever meant to be a fully accurate description of the reality but is intended to make complex science more digestible to those of us who find it largely inaccessible otherwise.

1. First, we have the ancient 'reptilian brain' dealing with the most basic functions of living such as regulating heart rate, breathing, digestion, body temperature and blood pressure. We share this with most vertebrates, and it is the part of the brain which is fully formed and functioning at birth in humans. It is made up of the brain stem and the hypothalamus and sits at the base of the brain, just at the top of the spinal column. If this part of the brain is damaged or malfunctioning, the person will be unable to survive without major medical intervention such as artificial life support.

2. Sitting above the reptilian brain, in the centre of the whole brain, we have the 'mammalian brain'. This part of the brain may have evolved later, as some animals evolved to function in groups and care for their young beyond birth. The mammalian brain comprises a collection of structures scientifically known as the limbic system. This is where emotions are processed, where we judge what is pleasurable or dangerous, and where we make snap decisions in the interests of our survival. This part of the brain develops in relationship with our primary caregivers in the first months of life and continues to grow and develop throughout the lifespan through our connections with others.

3. Lying above the mammalian brain we have the neocortex which is much thicker and more highly developed in humans than other mammals. The frontal lobes of the neocortex give us language and abstract thought, allowing for complex planning, communication, imagination, and creativity. An area known as the Medial Prefrontal Cortex, lying centrally, just above and behind the eyes, is particularly important in moderating our responses to trauma and stress. This part of the brain continues to develop throughout our lives through lifelong learning and connection with others.

These three areas work in harmony with each other to ensure our survival. Information enters our brain through our senses. Sensory nerves in our skin, eyes, ears, nose, mouth and inside our body detect stimuli in the environment and send that information to the limbic system in the mid-brain area for assessment. If the information looks harmless it is sent to the neocortex to be thought about, filed away, appreciated or dismissed. If the information looks worrying, it is rapidly sent to a tiny area within the mid-brain called the amygdala for urgent action. The amygdala is the early warning system of the brain, and it does not wait for further assessment before setting off the alarm and sending the troops into action. These 'troops' are the stress signals sent to the reptilian brain to increase heart rate and respiration and to release the stress hormones adrenaline and cortisol into the system to enable rapid fight/flight/freeze action. It is important to understand that rational thought is not involved at all in this stage of the process. The amygdala is activated instantly and triggers the response instantly. You don't get to decide rationally whether you will fight, flee or freeze, it happens automatically based on a very rudimentary assessment of the threat. The messages reach the thinking brain, the neocortex, much more slowly allowing us to then reassess the threat level and stand down the emergency response if it is deemed unnecessary.

Van der Kolk (2015) explains that in intensely emotional states the mid-brain areas become highly activated, whilst higher cortical areas, dealing with logic and impulse control, become relatively de-activated. In normal times there should be a balance between the activation of the early warning system and the oversight of the more rational brain, putting the brakes on the fight/flight/freeze response where it is not needed. Once the immediate threat is over, or the rational brain has deemed the threat to be non-existent, the body should soon return to its usual state of equilibrium. However, these processes are severely disrupted when significant trauma has previously overwhelmed the system, the slightest trigger may cause an intense overreaction, and equilibrium may not be regained so readily. It is as though the thinking brain is switched off and the autopilot of the reptilian brain takes over leading to loss of control and loss of awareness until the threat response subsides.

Why Did I Respond That Way?

This model of how the brain deals with trauma helps to explain some of the phenomena reported by trauma survivors. Some people report that during a traumatic event they acted in ways they are not proud of and feel a sense of 'survivor guilt'. One example might be a rail crash survivor who forced his way out of the wreckage, pushing children and old ladies out of the way to get to safety. He may look back with guilt and horror at his actions. Understanding that his rational brain was largely offline, and he was mostly acting from an instinctive fight/flight reaction can help to ease the guilt. Others report that they had previously thought they were strong and would fight off an assailant and so are deeply ashamed to find that they froze and 'allowed' a sexual assault to happen to them. Learning that fight/flight/freeze is not a rational, freely made choice but rather an automatic reaction can help shift self-blame and shame and facilitate recovery. In many instances fighting could worsen the outcome, fleeing might not be feasible, so freeze is the only viable option. As discussed in Chapter 3, the freeze/flop response has survival value and has evolved to give some protection even when things appear to be truly hopeless.

Neurobiological Impact of Early Developmental Trauma

The examples above assume the trauma survivor had a good enough early life, and this is the first trauma they have experienced. Research since the 1980s has shown that trauma during childhood affects the fundamental development of the brain structures involved in managing trauma. Dr Bruce Perry, a Child Psychiatrist in the United States, has studied and worked with traumatised children over many years and has shown that the absence of certain nurturing experiences, and/or the experience of various types of abuse, have significant adverse effects on the developing brain (Perry & Szalavitz, 2018). Having a caring, nurturing other, such as a loving parent, to help us regulate our emotions and understand the world is vital to our neurological development. Key parenting behaviours such as rocking and holding an infant, using baby-talk and singing help to wire their brain in such a way that they learn to comfort themselves. A parent who helps their child to manage big feelings by talking, comforting and modelling self-regulation allows the child's brain to wire itself so that they gradually learn to manage their own emotions as they grow. In the absence of good enough parenting, children do not learn adequate social or emotional skills and may exhibit anti-social or emotionally dysregulated behaviour. Alternatively, they will develop a tendency to dissociate, zoning out from the adversity and withdrawing from social connections. Behavioural difficulties and dissociation can in turn prevent a child from engaging adequately in education and social life which can lead to escalating exclusion, bullying and sanctions, which all serve to further traumatise the already traumatised young person. Sadly, children with these kinds of experiences may turn to bullying and anti-social behaviour, inflicting trauma on others due to their dysregulated emotions and lack of appropriate role modelling. Perry proposes a radically different approach for these children with his Neuro-Sequential Therapy process which strives to put back the experiences the child missed out on in a sequential way, mirroring the learning that would take place in a typical, good enough early environment and thus enabling the more adaptive brain wiring to develop. This can only happen once the child is in a safe and therapeutic placement, away from the abuse and neglect they have endured.

Perry's work with disadvantaged and traumatised children dovetails neatly onto Gabor Maté's work with addicts discussed in Chapter 5. It is the immense challenges of a traumatic childhood, Maté argues, that leads his clients into addiction, criminality and disease. If these children could be helped sooner, perhaps using Perry's methods, the societal burden of addiction, with all the health and criminal justice implications that go with it, could be reduced. Cuts to community services, social care and all types of healthcare are a false economy when we realise that more people are then left to follow the trajectory from traumatic childhood to mental and physical ill-health, addiction, criminality and so on.

The Importance of Supportive Others

Most trauma researchers agree that the effects of trauma can be mitigated by the presence of an attuned, supportive other. For young children this should ideally be the primary caregivers, as we get older they can be teachers, friends, co-workers or even a passer-by. Drawing on my own experience as an example, I did not have the most attuned or supportive parents. On a practical level, I was reasonably well cared for growing up, but emotionally it was something of a desert. When I nearly died in the hospital at 19 years old, it was not my parents who comforted me or reassured me but the hospital staff, from the cleaners and the ward clerk to the nurses, physiotherapists and doctors. I remember some of the staff to this day. Their words of support and comfort, their encouragement and kindness were new experiences for me. While my parents focused almost entirely on how much this catastrophic event had impacted them, the hospital staff told me I could build my life back, I could go to university, I could take up sport. They told me they could see my strength, my resilience, my intellect and my sense of humour. They had confidence in me and told me so. Without that emotional connection, I might have given up. Just one attuned, supportive other can reduce the impact of a traumatic event and set a person on the path to recovery.

Trauma and Neurodivergence

In Chapter 4, I mentioned that special consideration needs to be given to the interplay between trauma and neurodivergent conditions such as autism, ADHD and learning disability. This is an area that is under-researched and very hard to assess for a number of reasons (Mehtar & Mukaddes, 2011). These are lifelong conditions caused by a range of genetic, environmental and physiological factors. Autism is characterised by differences in social communication style, difficulties interpreting the thoughts, feelings and actions of others, a vulnerability towards emotional overwhelm, heightened sensitivity to sensory stimuli, having a narrowed range of interests, somewhat rigid thinking style and some avoidance of socialising. ADHD is characterised by difficulty focusing attention, over-activity, emotional dysregulation and difficulty either starting or finishing tasks due to distractibility and procrastination. Learning disabilities mean that the person is intellectually less able than most of their peers. These conditions will often co-exist with each other and with other physical and mental health conditions.

Neurodivergent people will often stand out as being different from their peers at an early age and can be significantly more vulnerable to experiencing victimisation, bullying and abuse than their neurotypical peers (King, 2010; Stack & Lucyshyn, 2021). One reason they will be more vulnerable to abuse is the difficulty they may have in understanding the intentions of others and reading situations accurately to assess risk, meaning that those with malicious intentions will have an easier job manipulating the neurodivergent young person. For example, a neurodivergent young person may naively accept those sweets from the stranger at the park and be led into a risky situation that a neurotypical peer might not. Once something has happened, the neurodivergent young person may have difficulty understanding or articulating what has happened, and even when they do, they are less likely to be believed or supported, especially if they are emotionally dysregulated when they attempt to seek help. Neurodivergent people who live in care settings are especially vulnerable to abuse due to the power imbalance between care user and care provider (King, 2010).

Assessment of post-traumatic stress in neurodivergent people is complicated by the overlap in typical signs and symptoms of these conditions (King, 2011; Stack & Lucyshyn, 2021; Brenner et al., 2018). For example, people who have been traumatised often isolate themselves for protection, whilst autistic individuals often isolate themselves due to feeling overwhelmed by social engagement. People who have been traumatised may find it very difficult to articulate what they have been through, and people with autism or learning disability may have difficulties with communication more generally. Similarly, both neurodivergent people and those who have been severely traumatised can display emotionally dysregulated behaviour. It is therefore complex to assess what is trauma and what is neurodivergence and needs specialist assessment. More research is needed on this complex area.

Trauma is likely to impact neurodivergent people more strongly than neurotypical people for several reasons (Stack & Lucyshyn, 2021). Deficits in information processing and problem-solving skills mean the neurodivergent person may struggle to use effective coping strategies. A tendency to be easily overwhelmed by environmental stimuli means that an event that is manageable to a neurotypical person may be completely overwhelming to a neurodivergent person. A rigid thinking style may mean it is difficult to think flexibly about what has happened and let go of unhelpful thoughts. Communication difficulties mean that reporting and processing the event through talking may not be possible.

Chapter Summary

- Neuroscience is complex, and we don't need a complete understanding of it to heal from trauma, but some knowledge can be helpful.
- Early neurologists did not have the benefits of modern technology to see inside the living brain but were still able to make helpful assumptions based on their patients' behavioural symptoms.
- The Triune Brain Theory is a helpful, if not entirely accurate, depiction of the key parts of the brain and how they function in the event of an overwhelming situation.
- Modern scanning technology enables more detailed tracking of brain processes during traumatic recall or viewing of disturbing video material.
- Understanding that our brains work instinctively to help us survive, rather than logically to act the way we think we should, can help us to forgive ourselves for seemingly irrational or inhumane behaviour in the face of overwhelming threat.
- Trauma early in life has a far more complex effect on the developing brain than trauma in adulthood. Bruce Perry and his colleagues provide training in his Neuro-sequential Therapy model to help those most adversely affected young people.
- We hope that by treating early trauma and its behavioural consequences, we can change the path that leads too many traumatised young people into the mental health and criminal justice systems.
- Just one supportive person can help significantly to mitigate the effects of trauma.
- Neurodivergent people are more likely to experience traumatic events, are likely to be significantly more adversely impacted by them and will struggle to use the coping skills neurotypical people would use.

7 Trauma and the Body

Medically Unexplained Symptoms

One rather contentious area in the study of trauma is the effect of psychological trauma on the body and on physical health. The adverse childhood experience (ACE) studies (see Chapter 4) describe the interplay between physical and mental health. Indeed, Freud discussed this in 1896 in his studies on hysteria. Symptoms of hysteria that Freud worked with included unexplained paralysis, unexplained blackouts, altered states of consciousness, unexplained physical sensations and pain. Nowadays some of these conditions might be re-labelled as Functional Neurological Disorder, Fibromyalgia, Somatisation Disorder, Complex Regional Pain Syndrome, Non-Epileptic Attack Disorder among others. Some of what Freud was seeing may have since been explained by progress in the medical field and the discovery of conditions that account for those symptoms. However, there remain many physical conditions that medicine cannot explain. For example, with modern brain imaging techniques, we can now differentiate between epileptic seizures and non-epileptic seizures; however, from a medical standpoint there remains a lack of understanding as to what causes non-epileptic seizures.

In the world of health care and mental health care, we tend to see a division between what is seen as the mind and what is seen as the body. You would usually go to a different hospital to see a mental health specialist than to see a physical health specialist. When something makes no sense medically, there is an assumption that it must be 'all in the mind', or even worse, a manipulative behaviour on the part of the person to gain attention. This all or nothing approach does little to help people with chronic conditions and can mean that where there is a psychological component to the condition, it may easily be missed.

Often what can happen is that once someone has a diagnosis of a mental health condition, any visit to the doctor with a physical health complaint that doesn't rapidly respond to pain relief or antibiotics will be put down to their mental health. People with mental health conditions often complain that their doctors do not take their physical health seriously. By the time they present to a psychologist, they are frequently very frustrated and resentful. This makes it very difficult to be helpful as a psychologist because the person will, not surprisingly, put up barriers and be unwilling to engage in any psychological work.

Mind and Body Are Intrinsically Linked

Since the 1990s, there has been a surge of progress in the field of trauma treatment using psychological therapies such as Trauma-Focused Cognitive Behavioural Therapy and EMDR (Eye Movement Desensitisation and Reprocessing Therapy). From this has come a greater understanding of the importance of a more holistic view of mind and body as being interconnected. Dr Peter Levine, a clinical psychologist in the United States, developed a model of trauma processing called Somatic Experiencing (SE). SE is based on the theory that psychological trauma is the result of incomplete actions leaving a residue of traumatic energy in the body. He explains this using the example of a wild prey animal being chased by a predator, it may freeze or flop but then if it manages to escape, it simply shakes off the experience and goes on with its day. Levine (1997) argues that humans tend to be thwarted in their attempts to shake off experiences and are compelled to relive them, thus perpetuating the trauma response. Trauma has very direct effects on the body, and these have begun to be studied in depth through the latter part of the twentieth and early part of the twenty-first century. Summaries of this work in the field of psychological trauma can be found in Babette Rothschild's book *The Body Remembers* (Rothschild, 2000) and Bessel van der Kolk's book *The Body Keeps the Score* (van der Kolk, 2015), both of which are based in the clinical and research findings of the authors, from working with traumatised individuals.

At the very simplest level, let's consider the impact that a stressful experience has on the body, such as an interview for a dream job or having an expensive new laptop stolen the day after buying it. Our mind and body interpret those situations as threatening, and we may experience a fight/flight type of response. Fight/flight, as we have already discussed, is a very bodily response as it is about physical protection or escape. As a one-off or very occasional thing, that is completely appropriate and is soon recovered from. The difficulty begins when the stress is chronic and/or severe and either there is no recovery time after one event before the next event occurs or a PTSD-type reaction occurs from which recovery is difficult without the correct support. We will all be familiar with the range of symptoms that such an event can bring about:

- butterflies in our stomach or chest area
- racing heart
- trembling limbs
- sweaty palms
- flushing face
- perhaps even an attack of irritable bowel or nausea

Our language also conveys the link between emotions and body sensations with the way we describe our emotional states – 'paralysed with fear', 'stomach in knots', 'flushed with embarrassment', 'flushed with success', 'jumping for joy', 'beaming with pride' or 'legs turned to jelly'. Our bodies are intimately involved in our emotional expression. The study of body language attempts to define what people are feeling and what is going on for them based on observation of their posture and movements. We take cues from how people hold themselves and respond accordingly. Someone in a power stance looming over us will elicit a very different response than someone cowering and turning away from us. Their body tells us something about their purpose or their level of confidence and triggers varying reactions in us.

Traumatic Stress and the Gut

One example of how chronic stress interferes with bodily systems is in the gut. Part of the fight/flight stress response is that the digestive system temporarily shuts down. The logic for this is that our evolutionary ancestors had to deal with very real threats to their lives, and there was no point in them wasting their energy digesting their breakfast if they were about to be breakfast for a pack of wolves. Far better to use those calories to run for the hills or launch a counterattack on the predator(s) or the invading hordes from over the hill. During fight/flight, all extraneous systems are temporarily put on standby so that energy and focus can be directed towards survival. If, once the threat is over, we take time to rest and digest, everything can go back to normal, and the smooth rhythmical flow of the digestive system can resume. This is true whether it is a real survival threat such as an assault or disaster situation or whether it is a more modern world threat such as work stress or a job interview. Either way, our mind interprets these as threats and the fight/flight response kicks in. If there is never a chance to rest and digest because one stressful event follows close behind another, then the gut can never settle back into its usual relaxed state of flow. This more than likely explains why so many people I have seen for therapy who have experienced trauma and adversity also experience gut problems such as irritable bowel syndrome.

Trauma affects all bodily systems, not just the gut. For example, if you break your shoulder in a car crash, the fracture may mend in about six to eight weeks, but the pain and tension you hold in that area may go on for much longer. This is partly because of how we tend to overprotect our injured area. We hold the area tense to prevent it from getting knocked, we avoid using the limb for fear of it hurting or doing damage, we may get an over-use injury somewhere else because we are guarding that area. These habits that set in soon after an injury become automatic very quickly, and we can continue overprotecting a limb without being aware that we are doing it. Hopefully after our car crash, we are sent to a physiotherapist who helps us to rehabilitate the limb, but in many cases, people live with chronic pain from injuries that have long since healed and make little sense medically. This is especially true where the origin of the injury is less clear, such as when the traumatic event was dissociated, and there is no recall of it. I have seen people with chronic pain in the pelvic region, which has 'always been there', which has resolved following trauma therapy during which they recalled a sexual assault, processed it and were able to let go of the tension that was causing the pain. This may seem extreme to people new to the field of trauma therapy, but it is not that unusual in clinical practice with trauma survivors.

Dissociation and the Validity of Memories

Dissociated traumatic events can be at the root of many 'medically unexplained symptoms'. There has been a lot of controversy over the years around the notion that people may recall things during therapy that were previously forgotten, and there have been accusations of therapists somehow implanting ideas in peoples' minds, or people making things up for attention or some other gain. The notion that these memories are always false has been challenged numerous times (e.g. Pope, 1996; Brewin & Andrews 2017), but the argument keeps on rearing its ugly head. In trauma therapy, it is not at all unusual for someone to be processing one memory and suddenly become aware of something else they had previously forgotten or been unaware of. What is striking is that it always takes the person by surprise, can cause considerable distress, but also makes complete sense and feels to them as though a missing puzzle piece has been found that makes sense of so many other parts of their life experience to date. This happened to me in my first Eye Movement Desensitisation and Reprocessing Therapy (EMDR) training workshop as I described in Chapter 2. As I was processing one innocuous event, an earlier, linked event came to mind, which then rapidly brought up another linked event which had previously been completely out of my awareness, as I had apparently dissociated from that event at the time and had never recalled it since, until that moment. Rothschild (2000) explains that some degree of dissociation is a defining feature of traumatising events and that it is unsurprising that dissociated aspects of a memory are held out of awareness, whilst other aspects, such as a bodily feeling or an emotional reaction, can remain. As with so many things it is important not to get too caught up in the binary of true/false, but rather to hold things lightly and see what emerges. An EMDR trainer I work with tells the story of a client who was convinced she had been raped by the devil as a child, but on further processing of the memory, it became clear that it was a relative wearing a Halloween mask. To the child-self, it had been the devil, but, on further processing, the adult-self recognised the child-self's simple error. Memory is not an exact science but at the same time we should never dismiss something just because it seems implausible at first sight.

In my own clinical experience, it has often been physical symptoms, such as blackouts, dissociative seizures or intense physical symptoms of fear that have led to breakthroughs in therapy. Whilst processing the physical symptoms, sometimes dissociated fragments of memory come into awareness, gradually making more and more sense to the person and presenting a clearer picture of what happened. As I stated above, I am not there to judge the validity of those memories but to help reduce the distress. Once the person has processed the memory and discharged the distress, the physical symptom typically reduces or even vanishes altogether.

When the Body Is Triggered

Once a person has some awareness of what is being triggered it becomes so much easier to make sense of bodily sensations and react with more compassion to their wounded self. A recent example for me as I write this chapter took place at my local gym. I had gone to swim and as I got out of my van, I noticed someone parking in an accessible space without a badge and looking extremely able-bodied, this was a gym after all. Obviously, I could not be certain that they did not have an invisible disability, but I wanted to challenge what looked like a blatant abuse of the disability parking space. I asked them if they had 'forgotten to display their badge', they grunted at me and went off into the gym. The receptionist overheard the exchange and told me she would put a warning on their vehicle. I went into the changing room and became aware of a severe trembling in my chest and a feeling of my heart racing as I replayed the brief interaction in my mind. It used to be very unusual for me to initiate a potential confrontation due to a fear of conflict instilled in me from a very young age by my aggressive father. For much of my life, I would have felt the injustice of the situation keenly but refrained from confronting it, and then I would have later regretted not saying something. Being so much more aware of my past now, I can separate out what is then and what is now. I was able to recognise that this was not my father, and I was not a small child. Therefore, I was able to speak up for myself as an adult in the situation. Then afterwards, as my body began to react, I was able to recognise that a part of me was frightened by my own actions, and I simply took a moment to soothe the frightened part of me before going on with my day. In the past, I might have either avoided the confrontation altogether and then been cross with myself for being a 'coward', or I might have said something, felt very anxious and then been cross with myself for being anxious, thereby exacerbating the uncomfortable feelings. Our aim in trauma therapy or in learning to cope with trauma is to learn to acknowledge the past, recognise that it is over and be kind to ourselves when having emotional or physical reactions to present triggers.

Body-Focused Therapy Approaches

The way I soothed myself in the example above was merely by placing a hand over my heart and speaking quietly to my frightened inner part. Simple physical actions like this can be very powerful in changing how we feel about a memory or a sensation. Some schools of trauma therapy, such as Levine's SE, focus very explicitly on the body and on the healing power of movement. Sensorimotor Psychotherapy is another such approach (Ogden, Minton, Pain, Siegel & van der Kolk, 2006). Noticing an urge to move in a particular way and carrying through with that urge can be a powerful intervention. For example, many times I have noticed trauma survivors jiggling their feet up and down during a therapy session when discussing a sense of being trapped or having no escape. I then encourage them to get up and move around or run on the spot and this helps them realise that they were trapped then but are free to move now, creating that vital separation between what was true then and what is true for them now.

In order to really notice the subtle movements and sensations in our body, we need to really slow down and focus on our bodily awareness. This is something many trauma survivors either actively avoid doing or really struggle to connect with. If physical pain was a part of the trauma you experienced, you might have learnt to dissociate from physical sensations and may now experience your body as mostly numb. When this has become a long-standing habit, it is very hard to reverse. Similarly, if noticing your body brings up feelings of shame or other reminders of what happened in the past, you may choose to ignore it and keep yourself distracted from it. Additionally, in our body-shaming culture, how many of us are truly comfortable enough with our bodies to really want to pay them that much attention? This is all entirely understandable, but not being in tune with the body means we don't take good enough care of ourselves, and we don't have access to the emotional signals that tell us which direction we need to go next. We will learn more about how to reconnect with our body and learn to read its vital signals in Chapters 12 and 13.

Chapter Summary

- Body and mind are closely intertwined and never more so than in the case of trauma reactions. *The Body Remembers* and *The Body Keeps the Score* are two key texts in the field of trauma that emphasise this link.
- Modern medicine tends to treat mind and body as completely separate, which serves to alienate those whose difficulties lie at the intersection of physical and mental health.
- Our guts are a vital indication of our overall well-being and tend to go awry when trauma strikes.
- Other physical symptoms are also a clue to past trauma and focusing on them may help to illuminate the past events, so that they can be understood and put to bed.
- We often find our body telling us it is scared or upset, we can soothe it with compassion and kindness, or we can beat it up with recriminations and harsh treatment. I wonder which approach works best!
- There are schools of psychotherapy that focus entirely on somatic (bodily) experiences and use movement and compassionate touch to relieve symptoms of trauma.

Part Two

Part Two

8 The Healing Journey

The Onion Analogy

I liken the process of therapy with trauma survivors to the process of peeling an onion. It's a metaphor I have heard many times, so I don't claim any ownership of it, and I have no idea where it originated, so I am unable to reference its creator. When people first come into therapy, there is often a reticence about opening up, based on fear and self-protection. This is like the tough outer skin of the onion. Anyone who cooks regularly will have had the experience of trying to peel and chop an onion, some onions give up their outer skin easily, while others are tough and unyielding and may need to be soaked in warm water to help ease off that outer protective layer. With some people, it takes a lot of gentle encouragement to break down that outer skin and reveal the layers beneath. In therapy, this is the process of building a rapport with the person, listening and helping them to make sense of their difficulties. Just to be clear, we do not typically soak our therapy clients in warm water to break down their outer layers of protection! We use compassionate listening, patience and gentle coaxing. Those who have had the most difficult experiences of life and of relationships will resist our attempts to understand and make sense, holding on tightly to the coping strategies they developed to get through the tough times and resisting any attempts to get them to try something different.

Unhelpful Coping Strategies

The coping strategies people develop to deal with trauma are many and varied, depending on their personality, their life experiences, their role models, the age at which the trauma happened and many other variables. It is important to note that people who have experienced trauma always did the best they could with the resources they had at the time. A child who learnt to dissociate and lose herself in fantasy as a way of avoiding the reality of an abusive parent is simply using her best available skills to hand at the time. That's what helped her survive, and we don't want to strip that away without offering something else in its place. Unfortunately, the coping strategies people develop within the context of early trauma are typically not the most successful strategies for getting qualifications, holding down jobs, making good relationship choices or generally coping with adult life. However, if these are their main strategies for coping with adversity, then of course they will be very reluctant to give them up or try a new way of coping. This is especially true if giving up those strategies causes memories and emotions from the past to emerge, intruding on the person's life and destabilising them. Tough onion layers need patience and care to work through.

Making Sense of the Problem

Often then, therapy is a process of carefully peeling away layer after layer to understand what lies at the heart of the onion, or the heart of the problem. An onion that has had favourable conditions to grow in, good soil, adequate water, not too many frosts or pests will be relatively easy to peel, and the layers will fall away without too much difficulty. Conversely, an onion that has had a more challenging start in life, many frosts, poor soil, pests and drought, may grow in a less regular way, with tougher outer layers, and may even have whole separate onions growing within it with tough skins of their own. When preparing onions, you sometimes find baby onions have formed within a larger onion. These more complicated onions require more careful processing because you have to take the baby onion out, peel it and chop it as if it is a separate onion in its own right, it takes longer and can be fiddly.

The person who has favourable growing conditions, good enough parenting, material comforts, safety and security but has then had a challenging event in adulthood will more than likely be one of those regular onions that doesn't take much peeling and is soon processed. Conversely, the person who has had unfavourable growing conditions early on, trauma, neglect, abuse, bereavement, abandonment, accidents or illness may present with a very tough outer shell and a complex series of 'inner onions' to be worked through before they are fully processed. This can also take longer and be fiddly!

The Three-Phase Protocol

Judith Herman first outlined a standard three-phase process for working therapeutically with trauma in her 1992 book *Trauma and Recovery*. Once the person has opened up a little to the idea of working through their trauma (the tough outer onion skin), Herman refers to a Stabilisation Phase (the next layer of the onion). This phase is about learning new skills for managing emotional disturbance. These new skills will gradually replace the older, less helpful coping strategies that the person has been using up to present. Once the person has mastered some of the skills of stabilisation and achieved some degree of emotional regulation, Herman states that they can move into Trauma Processing (there may be many onion layers to work through here, as well as some complete inner onions with their own tough skins). Trauma Processing can take many forms, it could be simply allowing yourself to sit and think about what happened, it could involve opening up to a trusted friend or family member, it could involve writing a book or journal about your experiences, or it could involve a period of formal trauma therapy with a suitably qualified trauma therapist. The third phase is what Herman refers to as 'Reconnection' and is less to do with the onion (or the trauma) itself and more to do with the dish you are going to make. Having processed the onions, how are you going to reconnect with the world and create a meal worth eating, or a life worth living, moving forward from the trauma? This might include finding new activities and learning new skills to live life with more sense of meaning and purpose, a change of career, or developing new relationships.

Do We All Need Therapy?

Much of this work can be done without engaging in formal trauma therapy. With the right conditions and some self-help guidance, many people can learn to live well with the aftereffects of trauma. In an ideal world, perhaps it would be a good idea for everyone who needs it to have access to good quality trauma therapy and to have the time in therapy to resolve all of their trauma fully, but often that is not realistic. There are many reasons why formal therapy is often not possible or realistic, for instance,

1. the statutory services are not available
2. services are available but there are long waiting lists
3. you don't meet the intake criteria for a particular service
4. private options are too costly for many people
5. life is simply too busy, chaotic and unstable right now to be able to engage in therapy

Maslow's Hierarchy of Needs

One of the foremost things we learn in psychology, and something you may have come across yourself, is Maslow's Hierarchy of Needs (Maslow, 1943), and it is always depicted as a triangle with a point at the top and a wide base. The triangle is divided into layers, showing our most basic needs at the bottom of the triangle, i.e. physical needs, then safety needs, moving up into more emotional needs such as love and belonging, then self-esteem and then moving up into higher order needs such as achievement and self-actualisation, i.e. living your best life. See Figure 8.1, Maslow's Hierarchy of needs (Maslow, 1943).

The purpose of Maslow's Hierarchy is to demonstrate that good foundations need to be in place before you can go on to 'self-actualise' or live your best life. What this means for self-development is that you need to have access to food, shelter, health and security, before you can really start to focus on learning, developing a career or resolving your trauma history. Simply put, if someone is in an abusive relationship, in insecure

```
            Self
        Actualisation

         Achievement

         Esteem Needs

        Emotional Needs

         Safety Needs

       Physiological Needs
```

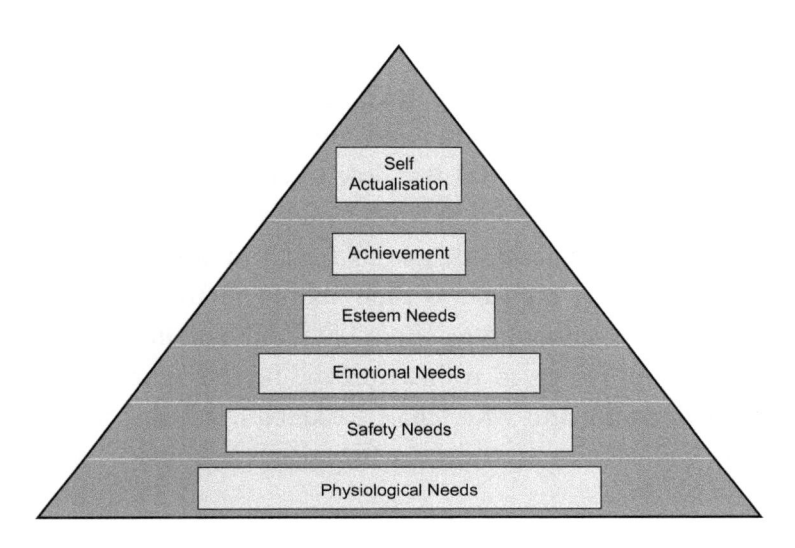

FIGURE 8.1 Maslow's Hierarchy of Needs.

housing, whilst trying to bring up children on a shoestring budget, they are not going to be in a mental space where they can focus on the higher order tasks of therapy or self-development. It will not matter how many well-meaning friends and professionals offer them self-help books or courses of therapy. At that point in their life what they need is support to establish safety, security and to meet their most basic needs. Over time, enough stability can be achieved for them to start working on the next stage of self-development, meeting their emotional needs such as the need for belonging and love, and resolving their trauma history. Self-actualisation may be a long way off for some people.

This needs to be understood at a societal level, so that social policy can be aimed at giving people the practical and financial support they need to ensure their safety and stability before they can put things in place to begin to escape poverty, heal their trauma and lead healthy, productive, satisfying lives. At a societal level, you can't force people out of poverty by heaping more trauma on them in the form of benefit cuts, unaffordable housing and a lack of social care support. All that does is trap people in poverty and inertia, desperately fighting to feed their children, or their addiction, but with no spare resources to progress in their lives.

I was fortunate as a young adult to have access to certain support mechanisms that enabled me to take my first steps towards healing from both my childhood trauma and my medical trauma. As a disabled person in 1980s Britain, I was able to claim certain welfare benefits that enabled me to afford to run a suitable vehicle, to rent reasonably accessible housing and adequately feed and clothe myself. With my basic needs being met, I was then able to focus on things that I enjoyed to regain a sense of purpose in life. I dabbled in various educational pursuits but struggled at that time to find the right thing for me. I took up swimming and wheelchair basketball, which I now believe were both invaluable in my recovery for several reasons.

How Do We Achieve the Right Balance in Life?

In Compassion Focused Therapy there is a model of living based around the balance between Achievement, Enjoyment and Connection with others. This is based on models of behavioural activation, originating in Cognitive Behavioural Therapy (e.g. Martell, Addis & Jacobson 2013). This can be depicted as a simple pie chart with the pie divided into three roughly equal segments representing the three areas of Achievement, Enjoyment and Connection, see Figure 8.2, The A-C-E Pie Chart.

Wheelchair basketball and swimming were activities that I took to very quickly and realised I could succeed at. This gave me a sense of *Achievement* which, frankly, having become disabled at 19 years of age, I really needed! At that stage, I was not sure I would be able to secure a job or return to higher education, particularly as there was no enforceable legislation at that time in the UK against disability discrimination. Both swimming and wheelchair basketball were also very enjoyable, there was a lot of fun and plenty of that good feeling some of us get after physical exertion, so I was getting *Enjoyment*. The other thing about both activities was that I was *Connecting* with other people who had some understanding of what was going on for me. In basketball particularly I was meeting people of all ages, many of whom were living well with disability – working, having families, studying – who could

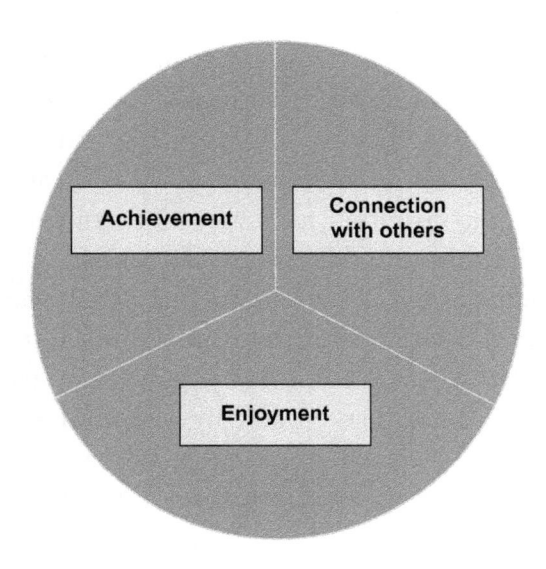

FIGURE 8.2 A-C-E Pie Chart.

be role models for me as I adjusted to my new life as a wheelchair user. So just with my sporting activities alone, I was already beginning to tick all the boxes in terms of building a balanced life. This then gave me a bit of a springboard to thinking about what more I wanted from life and how I might go about finding my way forward.

Sports and exercise might not be for everyone, but it is vitally important that we all find ways to meet the balance of Achievement–Enjoyment–Connection with others. It may be that you gain your sense of achievement from work, your sense of enjoyment from playing your violin, and your sense of connection from meeting with friends for meals out. There are an infinite number of ways to create this balance, for some people, this might be through their spiritual communities, through involvement in the arts, through community projects, through meeting others with similar needs (e.g. veterans groups, women's groups). For me, it was sport that showed me that my life was still worth something and that I could make a future for myself that could be very satisfying.

An additional point about connection that I want to make is that for some people, trust is so badly impaired that connection with other humans may have to be a more distant goal. When people have been let down and abused by everyone that should have taken care of them, it is not surprising that they would struggle to trust anyone. Many of these people have also been badly let down by healthcare services. Being shamed in the hospital Emergency Department for self-harming, being dismissed by the GP for 'attention seeking', being treated badly in inpatient settings, especially mental health wards. No wonder they don't immediately trust the next well-meaning person who comes along with a self-help book. For people where trust is so badly impaired, connection might need to start with connecting to nature, which is important for everyone, but more so for this group. Taking care of a few plants, sitting outside, walking in the park if there is one nearby might be important first steps. Alternatively connecting to animals might be a good next step. Caring for a pet can be very therapeutic and may help someone take those first steps towards healing. This may not be right for everyone, and pets do need to be well cared for, but it might be helpful for some people.

Often when people present for therapy, their coping strategies are focused on one area at the expense of other areas. Some might be prioritising Achievement, putting in many hours at the office to get the next promotion or pay rise, whilst neglecting their important relationships. Others might be prioritising Enjoyment in the form of drinking and partying to excess, whilst neglecting their career development. When Achievement, Enjoyment, and Connection with others are out of kilter, we tend to feel some dissatisfaction with life and need to find ways to get things back in balance (Gilbert, 2010).

Resources

By resources I mean the things we need in place before healing can occur. This includes such things as a supportive network of friends or family, a secure enough home, skills for self-soothing and self-care, meaningful activities, adequate income, food, and social care support if needed. A person who has had a good enough upbringing and is well-resourced will more than likely deal with a traumatic event much more easily than someone without those resources. The well-resourced person may be in the 75% or so of people who do not even go on to have a significant post-traumatic stress disorder reaction at all, even in the event of a horrific situation. If they do develop major difficulties following a traumatic event, they will be able to draw on all of those resources to recover much more easily than someone who lacks those resources. Over the course of my career, I have worked with people from healthy, nurturing backgrounds who have had lots of positive resources in their lives, including good relationships, hobbies and activities that give life meaning and satisfaction, jobs that give security and relative wealth, good self-esteem and self-confidence. I have also worked with people who lack all of that, people who have no social contacts at all, who are estranged from family, isolate themselves at home, cannot contemplate work or hobbies and have no sense of self-worth. The vast majority of people who present for therapy fall between these two extremes, and it is a matter of working out where their individual starting point for therapy and healing lies.

The better-resourced someone is, the sooner a therapist can get into the trauma work with them and the more likely they are to be able to work through their traumas with relative ease in a shorter timescale. The poorer the level of resourcing then the more work needs to be done to help build up those missing resources, frontloading them with the skills required to begin to face their traumas. A major part of my role is to help people learn some of the resources and skills they can develop to move them closer to being able to address their traumas whether or not they choose to do that through therapy.

Chapter Summary

- Therapy is a bit like peeling an onion. First, you have to get through any tough outer skin (resistance), then you have to process the multiple layers (of trauma), then you make the finished dish (a life worth living).

- Many people develop less than helpful coping strategies in the face of trauma, such as over-working, over-eating, over-thinking, drinking, shutting out emotion, avoidance of triggers.
- We need to learn new strategies for coping and let go of the less helpful ones.
- Trauma therapy typically happens in three phases – Stabilisation – Trauma Processing – Reconnection.
- Therapy is not always necessary, and people can do much to help themselves without therapy, but we must be mindful of how well-supported they are and what additional resources they may need to progress.
- We all need balance in our lives between Achievement, Enjoyment and Connection.
- Connection can be with nature and with animals as well as with other humans.

9 Helpful vs Unhelpful Coping

The Fine Line between Dysfunction and Coping

There is a very fine line sometimes between healthy coping and dysfunction. Some of what I am going to describe as coping strategies are healthy when used mindfully in moderation, but less healthy when used in excess or without mindful awareness. This situation can lead to confusion and is also a reason for some of the things we see on social media which are misguided attempts to be helpful. If we simply try to ignore our trauma and our feelings by distracting ourselves and putting a brave face on things, then those feelings are going to fester inside us and become more and more toxic over time.

Distraction

Much of the time, we do need to manage our emotions in order to behave appropriately or to get a task done. We learn early in life that it is not socially acceptable to throw ourselves on the floor of the supermarket and scream when we don't get our own way. From a very young age, we try to navigate the path between being overwhelmed by strong feelings and trying to become socially competent humans. One skill we may latch onto quite early in life is distraction. Parents will also use this strategy to manage tantrums in very young children, reinforcing the idea that distraction is a good thing and that giving in to feelings is something to be avoided. Indeed, distraction is a good thing, in moderation, when used mindfully. Watching a funny movie, going for a run, hanging out with friends are all great distractions when life is feeling a bit heavy. However, distraction alone will not resolve anything, it merely kicks the can further down the road. The challenge is to learn to use healthy distraction when appropriate, and alongside that, to process and express our emotions too.

Children use various forms of play and fantasy to distract themselves such as imaginative games, reading, computer games as well as TV and movies. Most of these activities present an alternative reality allowing the child to imagine themselves in a different or better world, with power and skills to conquer evil, for example. This is all part of a healthy childhood. However, when children are not being well cared for or are being abused, they have a greater need for distraction and that need may become problematic. Where a child feels powerless and helpless, losing themselves in fantasy worlds where they have magical powers to defeat the baddies is very attractive. Over time, we hang on to some of these more childish distractions but also add others to the mix.

Dissociation

Dissociation is an extreme form of distraction that happens automatically under extreme stress. This is often learnt in infancy if there is severe neglect and becomes the go-to strategy for all stressful events. It also happens in extreme events at any time in life, such as a sexual assault or being held at gunpoint. Dissociation is where the person's sense of reality becomes distorted or completely cut off. People describe time slowing down or speeding up, things seeming strange or unreal, a fogginess or darkness descending, sounds being muffled or echoing. If you are undergoing an extremely traumatic event, dissociation is protective as it acts like an anaesthetic. You don't feel anything and have little to no awareness of what is happening to you. If you survive the event, you may find you automatically dissociate every time the memory is triggered which makes it impossible to process the event and recover fully. You may only have a very patchy recall of the event, or even no recall at all.

Dissociation is automatic and does not resolve anything because it happens outside of our awareness. On the other hand, distraction can be a deliberate strategy to focus our attention elsewhere until we have a convenient time to reflect on what has happened. In learning to cope with trauma we are learning to take conscious control back so that rather than being at the mercy of our trauma and dissociation, we are able to ground ourselves, deal with what matters and use healthy distractions when needed.

Self-Inflicted Injuries

Sometimes in a dissociated state, or in a situation of extreme distress, people will injure themselves. The reasons for this are complicated and diverse.

1. It might be a simple distraction – 'I'm upset, if I hurt myself, I'll have something else to focus on'.
2. It might be a way of turning emotional pain into something more tangible – 'I'm upset, if I hurt myself, at least my pain becomes more real'.
3. It might help to ground them – 'if I hurt myself, it will snap me out of this mood'.
4. It might be that it inflicts the pain they feel they deserve – 'I'm stupid and made a mistake so I should punish myself'.
5. It might be a way of reaching out for connection – 'nobody cares, maybe if I have a physical injury someone will have to care for me'.

In any event, self-inflicted injuries are an expression of inner pain and reflect a need for support and connection. Punishing someone or rejecting them for hurting themselves will merely add to the weight of trauma they are carrying and ultimately cause more self-harm.

Self-inflicted injury is one of the least adaptive coping strategies that traumatised individuals come up with. Nevertheless, at the time, it is their best attempt to cope with overwhelming difficulty. These individuals need a compassionate space where they can be taught to stay more present and grounded so that the parts of themselves that want to hurt them don't get the opportunity to do so. This requires a patient connection with others who show unwavering care in the face of a very challenging and often alarming situation.

Substance Misuse and Dependence

As we get older, we discover new ways of numbing out and distracting ourselves. If we live with anger, hurt or sadness, we may very soon discover the soothing properties of alcohol and drugs to take the edge off our pain. Once again, there is a fine line between healthy use of substances and unhealthy substance misuse and dependency. Taking pain relief for a headache is usually a sensible thing to do. Having a glass of wine with colleagues on a Friday after work or with your partner over dinner is typically not seen as problematic, certainly in white, western cultures. While ever these things are done in moderation with mindful awareness, they may be part of a healthy lifestyle and help us to cope with trauma, stress and difficult feelings.

Dr Gabor Maté works with drug and alcohol-addicted people in downtown Vancouver, Canada, and has written extensively on the link between trauma and addiction (Maté, 2008). He describes how certain drugs, both medicinal and recreational, work by increasing the amount of feel-good brain chemicals at work in our brains. The brain chemicals Dopamine, Oxytocin and Serotonin all have important roles to play in driving our behaviour towards survival and all cause us to feel pleasure or calm when they are released in our brains. For example, Oxytocin is released in our brain when we enjoy sexual feelings, and when we nurse our infants, giving us a buzz of warmth and pleasure which reinforces behaviour aimed at reproduction and the survival of our young. Normally, once the brain chemical has done its job, it is collected and recycled by natural processes in the brain. Drugs of addiction block that re-uptake so that more of the feel-good chemicals are in circulation at any time. When the drug starts to wear off, the urge to re-use is strong as the fall in feel-good chemicals creates aversive feelings. The drugs of addiction are very well matched to the design and function of our nervous system, making all of us vulnerable to their effects. However, Maté

(2008) explains that genetic and environmental factors, such as trauma, exacerbate this vulnerability. In a healthy person, without a history of trauma, a strong painkiller such as morphine will help manage the pain of a broken limb, but once the pain is resolved, there should be no powerful urge to continue with the drug. In someone with a history of trauma, Maté argues, there is more likelihood of addiction developing because trauma alters the underlying brain chemistry.

Obsessional/Compulsive Behaviour

Often, we distract ourselves from trauma and unpleasant emotion by obsessing about other things. This might take the form of overthinking and worrying about everything. It might take the form of focusing excessively on cleanliness, safety or security. It might take the form of focusing excessively on body shape, diet or exercise. It might take the form of overworking. All of these behaviours are aimed at giving an illusion of being in control in an unpredictable world, distracting ourselves from the real problems we face and occupying our minds and bodies in ways that made sense when we started out but seem less logical once they have taken over our lives.

Again, there's a fine line that we cross at some point in our trauma journey. One day we are just distracting ourselves with a little extra study, towards getting into university and leaving behind the precarious existence of our youth. Over time we find it harder and harder to stop working and go home, because we are compelled to keep going by some irrational fear. One day we are reading a magazine or website as a distraction from the pressures of home life with overly critical parents, some time later we are obsessing about how to lose weight and achieve the proportions of the models in the magazine. It is as if, focusing deeply on that one thing will give a sense of control, security or safety that just seems to be lacking otherwise. What starts as a mere distraction from our inner emotional world becomes an obsession that is hard to let go of. Again, the more trauma we have experienced, the more likely these outcomes appear to be.

I would include here something which I have to hold my hand up to – obsessional scrolling of the internet. In evolutionary terms, this is a very new way of distracting ourselves and zoning out from what really matters. How many of us spend hours every week scrolling social media and news outlets, reading clickbait articles and generally wasting our time online? This is time when we could be connecting with our friends and family, getting our book written (yes, me again), or doing other things that might be of more value to us. One of the reasons this has become such a problem for us is because the designers of websites spend a lot of time and money researching what makes us tick, and therefore what makes us click. They have worked out how to make our brains release shots of dopamine to keep us clicking and scrolling. While they have us hooked, they can sell our attention to advertisers who create those annoying pop-ups that interrupt our scrolling experience. Arguably, the internet is a great way of accessing up-to-date news, information and keeping in touch with friends and groups we are linked to. Again, if we can keep it mindful and remain aware of when we are being led astray, it can be a healthy way of keeping in touch.

All of the obsessional behaviours can look very healthy at first. Overworking can look like conscientiousness. An eating disorder can look like disciplined healthy eating. Obsessional cleaning can look like being house proud. Over-exercising can look like good self-care. Scrolling the internet can look like staying informed and connected. In many cultures, these things are often highly praised, which can reinforce the behaviour and make it difficult to judge when it has gone too far. However, when they do go too far, they become extremely problematic, taking over our lives, creating enormous distress and keeping our attention away from the things that really matter. As always, the key is moderation and balance. If you are prioritising work, chores or exercise over everything else, worrying that you can't keep up, letting other things slip so you can do more of the obsessional activity then the balance has gone, and you may need help to regain that balance.

'Could Have Been Worse' – Minimising and Putting a Positive Spin on Things

The unhelpful coping strategies described above in this chapter can all be very harmful. Dissociation, self-injury, substance misuse and obsessional behaviours all get in the way of us living our best lives and can cause severe harm if left to escalate. They prevent us focusing on things that will make our lives feel fulfilled and worthwhile. They damage our relationships, our careers and our mental and physical health over time. At the slightly less harmful end of this spectrum we have a range of strategies that people employ that again create a distraction from the distress of trauma, and in the short term may even make us feel better. These strategies are all about minimising the issue or putting a positive spin on it. I would categorise these as the 'mustn't grumble' or 'could have been worse' group of strategies.

I have grown up in a largely white, western culture and throughout my life I have heard so many ways of minimising emotional distress. It may be a uniquely British thing – that stiff upper lip we were so proud of in the days of Empire and World Wars that still seems to be around. Phrases like 'man up', 'big kids don't cry', 'mustn't grumble', 'chin up', 'cheer up it might never happen', 'it could be worse', 'others have it worse', 'just look on the bright side' set up a culture where it is not considered acceptable to express our more difficult emotions. Those were the sort of messages I heard all around me growing up. Nowadays I see various iterations of these phrases all over social media, often with cheesy background photos of sunsets and beaches. I have to ask though; does it make my pain any less to know that someone else has it worse than me? Does it help me not to grumble? What if there is no bright side? What if I need to cry? I refer to this concept as toxic positivity. I did not coin the term myself, I don't know of its origin, but I have adopted it enthusiastically.

We know from decades of psychological research that holding in emotions causes them to fester and develop into mental health conditions such as anxiety and depression. We also know that unprocessed trauma stays locked in the mind with all the thoughts, feelings, images and body sensations from the time of the incident, and these are prone to be triggered by any reminder of the event (Shapiro, 2018). We need to process our trauma and express our strong emotions in order to regain balance and mental health. Minimising it, denying it and rationalising it away merely allows it to become toxic, infecting our thoughts, feelings and behaviour. To illustrate this with an example, I mentioned in Chapter 2 of this book how I recalled and processed a very early childhood memory whilst training in EMDR therapy. I recalled being hit by my father as a very young toddler. I had always been scared of my father and very angry with him and had not fully understood why until I processed that memory. As I processed that memory, I felt tremendous rage within me, which gradually dissipated as the processing went on. When I next visited my parental home, only a week or two later, I was noticeably less tense and anxious than I had ever previously been around him. Nothing else had happened in that time that would explain how differently I felt on that visit. That rage had been held within me for around four decades at that point and was always felt as a tense, angry, anxious sort of feeling when he was nearby. Resolving that took a considerable weight off my shoulders when I had to deal with him beyond that moment. He was still an impossible person, who brought up anger in me, but it felt very different. It was no longer the terrified rage of a hurt toddler, it was grown-up anger at an impossibly difficult person, which made it much easier to understand and express.

The Hierarchy of Unhelpful Coping Mechanisms

I tend to think of the unhelpful ways we try to cope in the form of a hierarchy from most harmful to least harmful. I think of dissociation as potentially the most harmful, as we cannot keep ourselves safe when we are so disconnected from reality. Self-harm and substance misuse come next in the hierarchy, closely followed by the obsessional conditions such as obsessions with diet/weight/body shape, overworking, overthinking, over-exercising. Last of all come the milder forms of distraction, minimising and positive thinking. This is a somewhat false hierarchy as it all depends on the severity of the presenting condition, but it gives an indication of how much we need to overcome in order to begin to make progress on actually facing and coping with trauma. If a person is at the more dissociative end of this spectrum, then they first need to learn to manage their dissociation through skills such as grounding and staying present in the here and now. If someone is using substances to excess, they may need medical help to detox and will need to learn new ways of dealing with difficult emotions. These steps will be easier to implement for those people whose coping strategies are less risky and damaging.

Chapter Summary

- There is a fine line between healthy coping strategies and dysfunctional behaviours.
- Ways we learnt to cope as children may not be serving us so well in adulthood.
- Dissociation, self-inflicted injury and substance misuse tend to be the most harmful coping strategies.
- There needs to be a balance between using coping strategies in a healthy way, whilst also acknowledging and dealing with our pain, versus becoming obsessively caught up in avoidance, distraction or minimising of our own experience.
- We need to learn to be mindfully aware of what is driving our actions, and when they are getting out of control.
- We are all starting from a different point depending on our experiences and the ways we have tried to cope so far.

10 Resources for Healing

What Do We Mean by Resources?

Before we can begin to cope and heal from our trauma, we need to do some groundwork to prepare us for the work ahead. I want to introduce some key concepts here that will help us to understand the task. The first concept is Resources, the second is the Window of Tolerance, and the third relates to the complex role of the Vagal or Vagus Nerve.

In the onion analogy described in Chapter 8, the onion that has favourable growing conditions does quite well in life and turns out to be well-rounded and stable in its construction. The same goes for a human with good growing conditions. As human infants are cared for and protected by their parents and wider community, they learn about themselves and internalise their experiences. Children who are loved learn that they are lovable; children who are abused learn that they are worthless. Children who are well cared for and provided for learn to care for themselves; children who are neglected learn to neglect themselves. Where the growing conditions are good, the child has the support and care to develop their own interests, building a sense of mastery and confidence in many things, including a sense of self-esteem. In a good enough family environment, a child will have internalised models of good self-care, self-esteem and self-confidence; they will develop interests that occupy them in positive ways and give them pleasure and satisfaction; they will develop wider social networks of friends; they will have the confidence to pursue career goals at whatever level is appropriate to their abilities. What I am describing here are resources – inner resources such as self-belief and self-esteem, and external resources such as friends, employment, leisure activities and family.

As discussed in Chapter 6, one important variation from the onion analogy is neurodivergent people. Neurodivergence is an umbrella term for people whose brains are wired differently from the majority (neurotypical people). This includes autistic people, those with brain injuries, intellectually disabled people and those diagnosed with conditions such as Attention Deficit Hyperactivity Disorder. Again, there is a vast range of experiences, but some neurodivergent people may be more powerfully affected by events that would not be considered traumatic by a neurotypical person even when all other aspects of their life have been positive. The difficulties neurodivergent people may face in life may both add to their experience of trauma and simultaneously impair their ability to manage the impact of trauma. For these reasons, neurodivergent people may require more support at all stages of life, most especially when they have experienced traumatic experiences.

Generally speaking, a neurotypical person who has had an adequate upbringing will be better resourced to deal with a difficult experience than someone whose childhood was lacking. If they do develop significant difficulties following a traumatic event, they will be more able to draw on those resources to recover. When dealing with trauma we are all starting from a different position depending on what resources we have and how our brain has been wired, or damaged. The fewer resources we start with, the more work needs to be done to build those resources as a first step to coping with trauma.

Window of Tolerance

The Window of Tolerance (Siegal, 2002) is a way of visually representing the zone of arousal within which a person functions best and is able to think, process and reflect on the situation they find themselves in. When someone is so overwhelmed by a situation that they have zoned out and cut off from the present moment, we say they are hypo-aroused (under-aroused). Other words for this state might include numb, frozen, depressed or withdrawn. When someone is in fight/flight/panic mode, we say they are hyper-aroused (over-aroused). Other words for this state might include anxious, angry, high-energy, overwhelmed or chaotic. There is a space between these two states where a person is neither over- nor under-aroused, where they can think clearly and see what is going on in the present moment. This space is called the Window of Tolerance (see Figure 10.1, Window of Tolerance).

Those who have had mainly good experiences and have developed healthy resources tend to have a wider Window of Tolerance than those who have not had the same advantages. Whereas someone who was abused or neglected will not have developed sufficient resources to cope and will have a much narrower Window of Tolerance. There will of course be a range of experiences in between the two extremes. Many people will find they need to widen their Window of Tolerance before being able to deal with memories and triggers relating to their past traumatic experiences. Even for someone who does not plan to process their trauma in therapy, it can be useful to consider ways to widen the Window of Tolerance simply to be able to deal more easily with the day-to-day stressors and triggers we all face.

It is likely that many neurodivergent people will have a narrower Window of Tolerance than most people. This may be because of an accumulation of unresolved past trauma, hyper-sensitivity to sensory

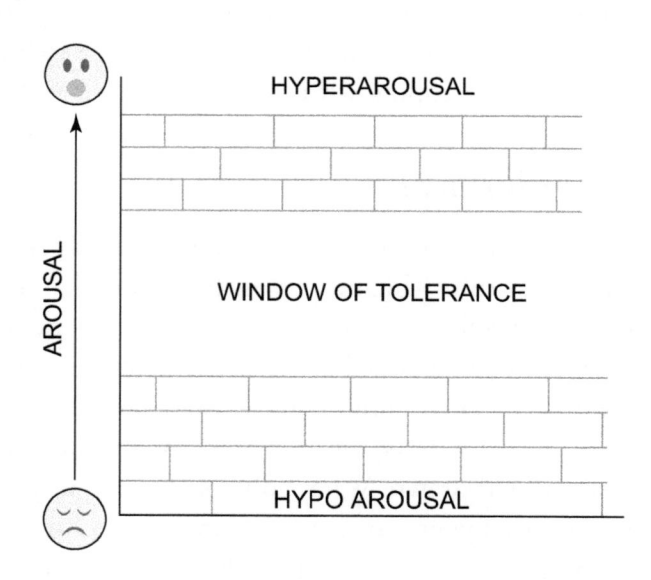

FIGURE 10.1 Diagram of Window of Tolerance. Source: Adapted from Siegal, 2002.

stimuli, difficulties asking for help or many other reasons. This may mean that more careful work needs to be done to widen the Window of Tolerance and address any barriers to accessing supportive resources.

The Vagal Nerve or 10th Cranial Nerve

The human nervous system is extremely complex. We have millions of neurons firing away in our brains, day and night, keeping vital functions working, controlling our bodies and interpreting our experiences. We have nerves transmitting messages from our body to our brain, and nerves transmitting messages from our brain to our body. There is much we still do not know about how our nervous system works, and much of what we do believe is based on theories, yet to be proven or disproven. Our understanding of the role of the Vagal Nerve, or the 10th Cranial Nerve has been important in theorising how our body manages our stress responses and how it keeps ticking over in the absence of stress.

Porges (2009) first introduced the Polyvagal Theory in the mid-1990s, see Figure 10.2, Polyvagal Theory: the Autonomic Ladder. His work built on the idea that we have a Sympathetic Nervous System which controls activation of the body in times of threat and a Parasympathetic Nervous System which regulates the body in times of calm or controls the shutdown of the body in times of extreme threat. These functions have long been known to be controlled by different branches of the Vagal Nerve or 10th Cranial Nerve. Porges expanded on this knowledge to introduce a third element, also controlled by the Vagal Nerve, which he named the Social Connection System.

The Social Connection System is controlled by a branch of the Vagal Nerve which leads from the brain to the front of the body around the face and throat and is called the Ventral (front) branch of the Vagal Nerve. In humans, this Social Connection System is highly sensitive and should be the first thing we turn to in times of threat. Ideally, we can call out for help and look for connection with trusted people to protect us. When the Social Connection System is activated, we should feel calm and safe, able to rest and digest and safely connected with

Polyvagal Theory: The Autonomic Ladder
Understanding the Nervous System
Adapted from Deb Dana, LCSW

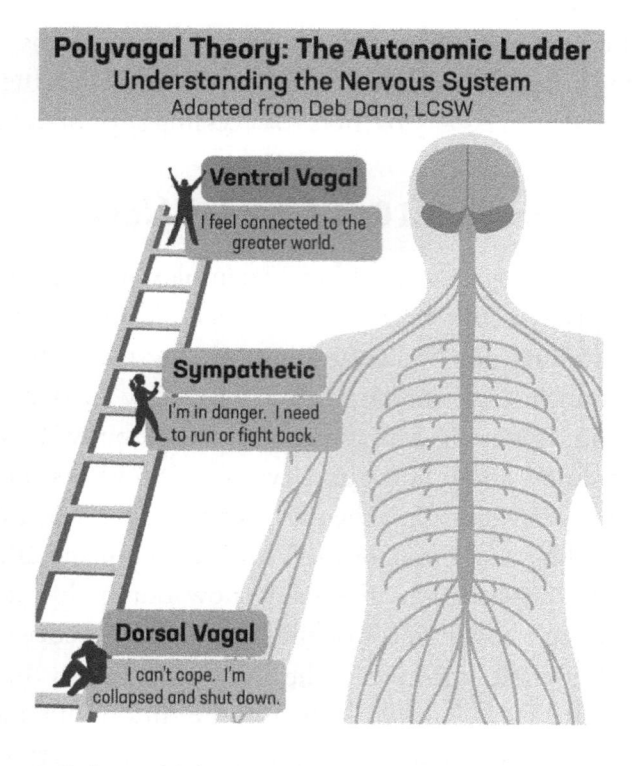

Ventral Vagal
I feel connected to the greater world.

Sympathetic
I'm in danger. I need to run or fight back.

Dorsal Vagal
I can't cope. I'm collapsed and shut down.

FIGURE 10.2 Polyvagal Theory: The Autonomic Ladder. Source: Adapted from Dana D, 2018.

others. If this fails and we feel threatened, we move into Sympathetic Activation (fight/flight), we try to flee or fight off the threat, with heart racing, fast breathing and adrenaline pumping. In a state of Sympathetic Activation, our thinking brain is less active, and our digestive system slows down or stops completely so that all energy and awareness can be focused on powering our muscles to fight or flee. In cases where we cannot fight or flee, we then go to the third option where we freeze or collapse, completely shutting down and feeling nothing. This state of collapse is controlled by the Dorsal (rear) branch of the Vagal Nerve.

Porges suggests that the most primitive response is the Dorsal Vagal shutdown which is common to all animals. This can be overridden by the more recently developed (by a few hundred million years) Sympathetic Arousal system – the fight/flight mechanism. This in turn can be overridden by the Social Connection System, a much more recent development in evolutionary terms and only existing in mammals, as far as we know.

Deb Dana (Dana, 2018) has written about the usefulness of Polyvagal Theory in therapy in teaching people how to gain control of their levels of mobilisation, disconnection and engagement. Dana describes these states as follows:

1. The Social Connection or Ventral Vagal state is a state of FLOW with feelings of being connected, engaged, peaceful, organised and at ease;
2. The Sympathetic Arousal or fight/flight state is a state of CHAOS with feelings of being out of control, overwhelmed, confused, angry, scared, mobilised for action;
3. The state of Dorsal Vagal shutdown is a state of DARKNESS with feelings of fogginess, darkness, numbness, hopelessness, disconnection, being shut down and immobilised.

When things are going well and there is no threat, we should be able to remain in the Ventral Vagal state, connecting with others and pursuing our life goals with ease. When a threat arises, we should go into sympathetic arousal (fight/flight) to deal with the threat and then easily return to Ventral Vagal state where we can rest and digest. When sympathetic arousal fails because we are alone, trapped or overpowered, we go into Dorsal Vagal collapse, our last-ditch survival mechanism. Again, if we survive the threat and live to fight another day, we return from Dorsal Vagal collapse to Ventral Vagal connection. The problem is that the more times we are faced with insurmountable or overwhelming threats, the harder it is to return to the Ventral Vagal connection state and the more we become stuck in chronic states of hypo- or hyper-arousal. In (Figure 10.2), the more times we fall down the ladder, the harder it is to climb back up again and the more time we spend stuck in states of hyper- or hypo-arousal.

When we have experienced traumatic events, our mind and body brace themselves for further trauma. We remain hypervigilant, on edge, looking out for danger, and we are very quick to enter the fight/flight state at the slightest hint of further threat. When we have experienced serious, chronic trauma, where there has been no possibility of escape, we are very quick to go straight into the freeze/collapse response. Therefore, survivors of trauma typically feel out of control and may even wonder if they have lost their rational minds. For those of us who have had poor experiences growing up, whose needs have not been adequately met or who have had no trusted others to rely on, the Social Connection System will not be robustly developed and may easily be overridden by more primitive responses of fight/flight and freeze/flop. Whereas for those of us who have had a good enough experience of growing up in a loving, safe environment, our Social Connection System will be well developed and will be the first system to engage when a new threat looms. This will help us to assess the level of threat more mindfully and override the fight/flight and freeze responses in all but the worst of situations. If we wish to have more control over our responses, to feel less threatened by everyday experiences and to develop a more satisfying life, we need to retrain our Vagal Nerve and build a more robust Social Connection System.

What Do We Need to Heal from Trauma?

1. *People*

It is not simply a matter of how much trauma a person has experienced, but also, how much they felt supported by caring others, either during or after the experience, that will determine how severely they are affected by it. Humans are innately social creatures who historically needed the support of our community to ensure our survival. A traumatic event endured alone will therefore have a far more devastating impact than the same event experienced in the presence of empathic, supportive others. Part of our healing journey will require us to find new people we can connect with, especially if we are estranged from our friends and family of origin.

There are many ways of finding our people, but for those who have been through trauma, this can be fraught with difficulty. Typically, people meet through education, work, hobbies and social events. If your trauma experiences mean you have withdrawn from these activities, then it will be more difficult to find that connection. Not surprisingly, those who have been harmed by others in the past struggle to trust new people and therefore shy away from forming new connections even if they do engage in activities. Negative self-beliefs, learnt through traumatic experiences, can also be a barrier to connection with others. Fears about the world being a dangerous place can mean that those who have experienced trauma avoid going out into the world, and thereby miss the opportunity to connect with new people. If we are to find our people, we have to overcome these barriers, and I will discuss ways of doing this in subsequent chapters.

2. *Knowledge*

I very much hope that if you have read this far, you are already gaining an understanding of why you feel the way you feel. Knowledge is a powerful thing. Without knowledge of how trauma impacts us, we can easily think we are going mad, that it is our own fault or that we deserve to feel bad. Once we understand that our Vagal Nerve is trying to protect us, that our Window of Tolerance is narrowed by our experiences of trauma, that our system automatically shuts down or goes into overdrive when we are triggered or threatened, we can start to think more kindly towards ourselves. This includes forgiving ourselves for our natural reactions and moving more easily towards self-care and healing.

3. *Skills*

There are many skills and exercises we can practice to gain mastery over our nervous system and release ourselves from the automatic reactions that cause us such distress at times. We need to learn ways of keeping ourselves mindfully present and grounded to counter the effects of unnecessary hyper- or hypo-arousal, see Chapters 12 and 13. We need to train our nervous system to keep us more engaged and connected, see Chapter 13. We need to learn to manage our unhelpful thoughts, see Chapter 14. We need to find new activities to build on these skills in our own time, as we move towards healthy coping, see Chapter 15. We also need to learn self-compassion and develop skills and resources around being kinder to ourselves, as this is a vital part of healthy coping, see Chapter 14.

Chapter Summary

- If we have had a good enough start in life, we more than likely have good resources for dealing with adversity when it happens. If not, then we will need to build up new resources in order to begin healing.
- Neurodivergent people can be more susceptible to the effects of trauma even when they have been well supported in early life as discussed in Chapter 6.
- The Window of Tolerance refers to the zone in which we can be rational, connected and effective in our actions, in between hyper- and hypo-arousal.
- The vagus nerve has important roles to play in moderating our responses to trauma and can be trained to respond more helpfully in the face of threat.
- If we are to cope and live well with the trauma, we need the right people, knowledge and skills.

11 Acceptance and Commitment Therapy

Acceptance and Commitment Therapy – A Model of Therapy and an Approach to Life

I cannot go much further into this book without referencing the work of Dr Russ Harris, a therapist, writer and trainer who has influenced my parallel journeys of self-healing and professional development in equal measure. Harris has written extensively on Acceptance and Commitment Therapy (ACT) and has shared much of his own journey dealing with trauma and anxiety in his writings and teachings. His book *The Happiness Trap* (2007) is one of my most common recommendations to people at the beginning of their healing journey as it gives such an accessible explanation of what it means to be human and to deal with the complexity of having human emotions.

ACT (pronounced as a word 'act', not as the three letters A-C-T) is a model of therapy that has really gained traction since the turn of the twenty-first century in western psychotherapy. ACT draws on the best of many therapy traditions, as well as drawing heavily on eastern philosophical traditions. The aim of ACT is to help develop greater flexibility of thinking to enable more flexible ways of responding to the world around us. For example, if our response to stress has always been to drink alcohol, this may, more than likely, have led us into difficulties at times. Developing more flexibility opens up new choices of how to respond to stress, for example by learning to meditate, or using healthy exercise. At its most basic level, ACT teaches us how to be more present in the moment, more open to our emotions and more focused on acting in the service of our values.

ACT is known as a third-wave Cognitive Behavioural Therapy (CBT). Traditional CBT encourages us to focus on our negative thoughts and feelings and work on strategies to banish them. However, ACT takes a different view, finding that if you focus on the negative thoughts and feelings and get into a struggle with them, then it perpetuates the negative thought or feeling rather than reducing it. To elaborate with an example, imagine you are stuck in traffic, you are in a rush and you want to get to your destination, so you look at the traffic ahead, you try to calculate how long you will be stuck, how late you will be, and your frustration mounts. You might rev your engine, beep your horn and thump your dashboard in anger. None of which resolves the fact that you are stuck in traffic, all it does is raise your blood pressure and put you into a state of hyperarousal, outside of your Window of Tolerance. You might then beat yourself up for being so impatient and angry, thinking about all the times you've lost your temper in such situations before, and feeling shame and anger with yourself for having these feelings. Again, this only makes you more frustrated and pushes your blood pressure higher. If only you could look at the traffic, acknowledge that you will be late and note that while it is frustrating, it is not the end of the world, you might be able to arrive at your destination, late, but in a reasonable mood considering.

How I Applied ACT before It Had Been Invented

Drs Steven Hayes, Kirk Strosahl and Kelly Wilson first wrote about ACT in the late 1990s (see Luoma, Hayes & Walser, 2007), so ACT had not, strictly speaking, been invented when I became disabled as a 19-year-old. Nonetheless, looking back there were elements of ACT playing out in how I chose to live my life even way back in the late 1980s. I think I very quickly realised that some things just cannot be denied, I had lost both legs and was never going to be able to walk, but I had a sense that there were people out there living fulfilling lives as disabled people. So even whilst going through a deep grieving process, I was already looking out for ways to live a meaningful life again and making whatever adaptations I needed to be able to do that. Even whilst still in the hospital I had a conversation with one of my physiotherapists about wheelchair basketball as I had heard it was 'a thing'. She confirmed it was indeed a thing and said she could introduce me to the then-captain of the GB men's wheelchair basketball team as she was also treating him for a shoulder injury. This was how I came to be introduced to Sir Philip Craven MBE who later went on to be president of the International Paralympic Committee and who, back in late 1986 to early 1987 – took me along to a few wheelchair basketball training sessions and got me hooked on the sport. In ACT, the emphasis is on accepting the present reality, whatever that may be, opening up to the emotions that are there, whether good, bad or neutral, and taking steps in the direction of our values. I accepted the loss of my legs, I grieved for that, and I strove to make a meaningful life for myself beyond that. I did not apply ACT fully, after all it had not yet been written about, I was not yet a psychologist, and I was just running on instinct back then.

Experiential Avoidance

It is fair to say that those of us who have experienced significant trauma in our lives do rather tend to avoid sitting with our innermost thoughts and feelings for long. When we feel neglected or abused by our caregivers as we grow up, the last thing we want to do is dwell on how awful that feels. When we have lost limbs, or experienced some other major life event, the tendency is to move away from thoughts or feelings about it. So, we learn strategies to distract and avoid those deeper experiences. Gabor Maté's patients in downtown Vancouver did this through the use of drugs and alcohol, others of us do it through distraction, overworking, obsessional thinking, among other ways. In ACT this is labelled 'Experiential Avoidance', and it becomes a well-practiced habit that is very hard to break. For myself, I found that throwing myself wholeheartedly into studying, sport and work meant I did not stop still long enough to really feel much about my earlier trauma. Despite pragmatically accepting what had happened to me, I still carried an awful lot of emotional baggage with me from the past for many years well into adulthood, rarely stopping to assess the load, or shed any of it. However, through my studies, I did learn new skills and was able to become more flexible in how I dealt with my past. As I have progressed in my profession, I have also used psychological therapy from time to time, to begin to break down my Experiential Avoidance and confront my past. This is not a 'one and done' process for me. Rather, I view it as a journey, with many stops and detours along the way. Some of those stops and detours are very much based in avoidance. At times I confront my past through therapy and at other times, it is just necessary to take a break, get on with normal life, avoid the reality and come back to it later.

This is the fundamental choice for trauma survivors – to avoid or confront. Herman (1992) called it the Dialectic of Trauma – healing can only really come from opening up and confronting the past, but our most basic urge is to avoid it at all costs. Harris (2019) introduces us to the idea of every moment being a choice point. The choice being, on the one hand, to react in our usual way to whatever is happening, perhaps with Experiential Avoidance (in the form of overactivity, over-thinking, distraction, numbing out, overeating, self-harm or substance misuse) or, on the other hand, to notice mindfully what is happening and make a conscious choice to take a step in the direction of something that makes life meaningful. Moving towards the things that make life meaningful, even when life is proving difficult, means that we do not get too bogged down in the difficulties and are able to have a satisfying life, while accepting the challenges we face. This is far from easy when you have experienced a lot of trauma and are well-skilled at avoiding, but it is something that can be learnt and developed with practice.

When Is a Coping Strategy Just Another Form of Avoidance?

To expand on my example above from my personal experience with trauma, having become an amputee wheelchair user I had little choice but to accept the reality of the situation. I felt the physical and emotional pain as I grieved that loss AND I got on with finding new things that would give me a sense of purpose, satisfaction and direction in life, such as sport and study. I quickly realised that my parents were not a great resource to support me in this and sought out a new community for myself initially in the world of disability sport and then also in academia and Psychology. There is a fine line between what is a resource, a coping strategy or an act of avoidance. At times the same action could be any or all of those. For me, I think I was driven into taking up certain activities as a way of avoiding some of the inevitable pain of what I had been through, but they became useful resources because they were fundamentally quite healthy things to do, in moderation. I'm not so sure I always kept things in moderation and was always striving to prove myself in the early years of my adulthood. The striving and the proving myself has led me to be successful in my various fields of endeavour; however, I do sometimes look back now and wish I had put less pressure on myself and taken more time to simply enjoy the journey!

As discussed in Chapter 9, there is a fine line between helpful and unhelpful coping strategies. For example, you might see a glass of wine as a pleasant reward to help you unwind at the end of a hectic week at work, enjoyed with a nice meal every now and then. Nothing wrong with that of course, in moderation, for most people. But what about when that nice relaxing glass of wine becomes two or three glasses, maybe quite large glasses, maybe five to six nights a week, until you start to realise you can't get through the week without consuming a substantial volume of alcohol? Then it becomes an unhealthy coping strategy, rather than a helpful resource. It becomes a dependency, a way of numbing out and avoiding whatever the present moment holds for you. Whatever we do to cope, we need to be mindfully aware of how much we are depending on that strategy to get through and whether it is kept in healthy moderation.

Acceptance versus Toxic Positivity

Whilst this is not a book about therapy for trauma, but rather a book about how to cope with trauma, it is useful to know a little about the various approaches used in the treatment of trauma. I bring in ACT here as it is such a useful way of thinking about life, about being human and about how we deal with our difficulties. Over the last decade or so, since I have really begun to understand ACT in some detail, it has become deeply intertwined with how I live my life and how I interact with the people who come to me for therapy. My very favourite thing about ACT is how it stands firmly against something I have long disliked in Western Culture, something I, and many others, refer to as 'toxic positivity'. Toxic positivity is everywhere, especially on social media. It is very hard to open up any social media platform without seeing some idyllic picture of a sunset and some cheesy quote about everything happening for a reason, or how a smile and a positive attitude will make everything alright. It is simply not true. Some things happen that make no sense, child abuse for example, simply should never happen, there is no rhyme or reason for it. A positive attitude will not make racism or misogyny or ableism go away. And a positive attitude certainly won't make cancer go away. I have lost friends to cancer at young ages, and there is no bright side to it. There is no sense to this, and no amount of positive thinking or reassurances will change it, it is horrible and that is all there is to it. ACT takes this stance, it's horrible, let's acknowledge that, let's feel all the feelings and then let's get on and do whatever we can in the face of it in line with our own personal values. In fact, ACT states that trying to deny the difficult stuff and push away 'negative' emotions simply makes things worse. The more effort we put into pushing away difficult feelings, the more our focus is on those difficult feelings. The more we battle them away, the more they intrude into our life, overwhelming us and making things worse than they need to be. We need to let go of the struggle, notice what is really there, open up to it and get on with what is important to us.

One way I put this into action back in the 1980s was with my rehabilitation from meningitis and amputations. From the moment I woke up in the hospital, I kept being reassured that I would walk again and that modern prosthetics would be the answer. It seemed like there was an expectation that I would want to strive to walk again and not be 'confined' to a wheelchair (as if that is such a negative thing). At first, I bought into this ideology, I went along to the limb centre and got fitted for a pair of above-knee prosthetic legs. They were big, cumbersome, unwieldy, heavy things that looked nothing like the real thing and worked even less like the real thing. They were also exceptionally uncomfortable. For a while I pursued this aim of learning to walk and had new better legs made and spent several days every week at the physiotherapy department, swinging up and down between parallel bars, in a sort of pseudo-walking motion. I made some progress, but simply could not balance outside of the parallel bars. I had no strength in my lower body, and no amount of practice seemed to improve that. Rather than take the ACT approach, the physios and doctors just felt I should try harder and longer and somehow the miracle would happen. However, I very soon had different ideas. I was a 19-year-old woman, just starting out on adulthood, and I had things to do, people to meet, places to go! I rapidly decided that I did not have time to spend my entire youth parading up and down the parallel bars of the physio department. I was seeing full-time wheelchair users at basketball living their lives very well and I realised I did not have to learn to walk. I could continue to be a full-time wheelchair user and free up all that physio time to do things that would make my life more meaningful, like sport and work and study. Had I listened to the advice I was getting from the medical professionals at that time, I think I would still be there now, swinging up and down between the parallel bars, trapped in a world of trying to learn to walk, growing increasingly frustrated and disappointed. Whereas my decision to leave all that behind and take on life as a full-time wheelchair user was the liberation I needed and has served me well. I have been free to live my life, my way and have achieved rather a lot, though I say so myself. In accepting my reality, I freed myself up to really live my life.

Chapter Summary

- ACT has been around since the 1990s and is a very different approach to mental distress than some other approaches. Rather than focusing on identifying and removing negative thoughts and feelings, it encourages us to engage with them and accept them.
- ACT emphasises being mindfully present with whatever is, in this moment. We then use this mindful awareness to make a choice as to how to proceed – follow our usual habits or take a step towards our values?
- Often, our usual habits have been in the service of Experiential Avoidance rather than our values. ACT encourages us to let go of toxic positivity and really get to grips with reality, however gritty it may be right now.
- There's a fine line between healthy and unhealthy coping strategies and between acceptance and giving in. We need to stay mindful to know which is which.

12 Mindfulness

Mindfulness

The first step in being able to make those more helpful choices is to learn to notice what *is* in the present moment. What is real, what is happening, what's the reality for me right here right now? Present moment awareness is a fundamental skill to be learnt in the service of self-healing. I first learnt about mindfulness as a newly qualified Clinical Psychologist back in the mid-1990s. It wasn't something I had been taught in my training, which seems almost unbelievable to me now as it is such a fundamental part of my work nowadays. Mindfulness is about being fully aware of the present moment with acceptance, non-judgement and compassion (Kabat-Zinn, 1996). I had been to a workshop on self-compassion and Compassion Focused Therapy led by Professor Paul Gilbert, who, a few years later, published his ground-breaking book *The Compassionate Mind* (Gilbert, 2010), and I had been intrigued by the idea of mindful meditation. I came away and researched the idea, looking for guided meditation resources to begin a mindfulness practice of my own.

My research led me to two inspirational teachers, first Professor Jon Kabat-Zinn and, through his writings, Thich Nhat Hanh. Kabat-Zinn is a Professor Emeritus of Medicine, Massachusetts, USA. Kabat-Zinn has developed and used mindfulness practices, both personally and professionally, to benefit himself, his cancer patients and also health care practitioners and the wider public. His teachings help people to manage a multitude of stressful situations, from terminal cancer and the horrific pain that can go with that to everyday workplace stress and strain. In his writings, Kabat-Zinn refers very lovingly and reverently to the late Buddhist Zen Master Thich Nhat Hanh (1926–2022), who was a Buddhist monk exiled from Vietnam to France during the Vietnam War. Thich Nhat Hahn, known to his followers as Thay (teacher), has brought Buddhist teachings on mindfulness to a wider western audience through his writings and the practice centres he set up across the world during his long life. It is important to emphasise that you do not have to become a Buddhist to appreciate his teachings, and also that mindfulness is not a religious practice that will in any way interfere with your existing beliefs or spirituality. It is simply the act of paying focused attention to the present moment, right here, right now, whatever that moment consists of, whether it be good, bad or indifferent. You do not even need to meditate to achieve this. Many people struggle to meditate, and it really is not essential.

At the point where I was discovering mindfulness, I had just turned 40, just qualified as a Clinical Psychologist and had a six-year old child with disabilities to parent. This was, in fact, a relatively calm period in my life compared to the preceding 20 years of frenetic activity. I had spent much of my 20s and 30s running away from the multiple traumas of both my childhood and the meningitis I had experienced at age 19. I had thrown myself headlong into wheelchair basketball and had an international playing career there, whilst also getting back to studying, completing my degree and embarking on the journey towards Clinical Psychology training. Simultaneously, I was getting married, having a child and all that came with the early parenting of a child with multiple difficulties. It is fair to say that as things began to slow down, I became quite agitated and stressed, almost wanting to look for the next challenge, and the next, to keep me from stopping and noticing anything deeper than what was on the surface of my awareness. However, by this time I was reading Kabat-Zinn and Thich Nhat Hanh and listening to audio tapes of guided mindfulness meditations. I began to lean-in to the agitation and just notice it. It was not easy. My entire being wanted to avoid the process, and it still does to a lesser degree. I resisted and fought with myself on a daily basis. 'I should listen to a guided meditation', I would think, 'but first I'll just tidy the kitchen, do some gardening, play with my kid, scroll the internet, anything but focus on me and my inner world!'. Even now, many years later, I still struggle to prioritise meditation, but the difference now is that I can accept that resistance with compassion, and then, at least sometimes, do it anyway.

There are many ways of getting present. Formal mindfulness meditation practices are a good introduction, using smartphone apps and recordings from the internet can be useful. Be aware though there are so many out there that it can be difficult to choose and as always with the internet, some are simply rubbish. Always ensure you like the product before you part with any money or sign up for a subscription. I still use guided meditations intermittently as they can be helpful in calming the mind when stress is taking over. Apps that I recommend and use myself are listed in Chapter 16.

Less Formal Practices for Mindfulness

I have also found ways of being mindful that are not necessarily about formal meditation but are more to do with meditative activities. Most days now I swim in the morning, I go to the same pool, maybe 4–5 times a week, and swim up and down for about 30-45 minutes, thinking of very little indeed, letting my mind roam if it needs to, but mostly just focusing on the feel of the water, the sensation of my arms moving, the rhythm of my breathing. Most weekends I will find an open-water swim session to go to. This is a relatively new activity for me, I began in the summer of 2021. Frustrated at the repeated closure of the gym over the preceding year due to the coronavirus pandemic, a friend introduced me to an organised outdoor swim session where it felt accessible and safe. I was immediately hooked and have continued swimming right through the winters here in the UK, where the temperatures in the water can go down as low as 2–3°C. It can go colder, but I have my limits! It is important to be aware of the risks as well as the benefits of cold-water swimming. I only swim at organised sessions, where there is safety and supervision available. Most venues offer an induction to new open-water swimmers covering the key safety points and risks to be aware of. Nevertheless, there is something about getting into a cold lake in the middle of the countryside that really brings you back to yourself, you cannot help but notice the sensation of ice-cold water on your body, even in a wetsuit. Equally, the sense of a deep connection with nature and the social connection that happens incidentally at these swim sessions adds to the overall sense of pleasure and reward that comes from this activity.

You do not need a pricey gym membership to use exercise for mindfulness. You can walk mindfully, run mindfully, cycle mindfully. If safety is a concern for you, as it is for many people, particularly people who have experienced trauma, finding an organised group activity or at least a buddy to do the activity with may be vital. If that is beyond your ability or comfort zone for now, there are many home-based exercise routines you can access through the internet. During the first UK lockdown of the Coronavirus pandemic in 2020, I found several yoga classes on YouTube which were free and could be done in the privacy of my own home. I was having some issues adjusting to online work, and my neck and shoulders were constantly screaming at me due to poor posture at the computer. Free to access online yoga classes aimed at loosening up the neck and shoulder areas were transformational for me at that moment. I am no expert in yoga, and without legs I am not really built for many aspects of yoga. Nevertheless, yoga is a practice rooted in mindful eastern philosophies, and it is well regarded in the treatment of trauma as a way of reconnecting mind and body and relieving physical symptoms of emotional trauma. A ten-minute neck and shoulder workout probably isn't going to heal your trauma, but it may be a gentle introduction to a form of exercise that you might be able to take further through classes as your confidence builds.

Creative Practices

For people who are less attracted to physical activity, there are many creative pursuits that also help to develop mindfulness skills and present moment awareness. This is where the clichés of having a relaxing bath or colouring a picture come in. Nobody should be suggesting that having a nice bath or doing a spot of colouring will heal your trauma or resolve a mental health crisis. If anyone is suggesting that then they have missed the point entirely. However, these activities, and many others such as crafting, baking, gardening, making pottery, almost anything you can think of really, can help you to develop the skills of present moment awareness and concentration that will help you to take the next steps in opening up to your emotional inner world, and maybe even facing your traumatic memories. At home, I have a book full of meaningless geometric patterns and a set of colouring pencils and every now and then, as a way of training my mind to focus on one activity for an extended amount of time, I do a bit of mindful colouring. When I do this, I am immediately aware of voices in my mind telling me not to go over the lines, criticising my choice of colours and telling me it needs to be perfect or it's no good at all. I know where these voices come from, they are the internalised voices of my parents, for whom nothing I did ever seemed good enough. For much of my childhood and early adulthood, I simply could not apply pencil to paper in an activity like that as I would be so tense and afraid of getting it wrong. Practicing mindfulness has taught me to notice that and respond with acceptance and compassion, so that now when I pick up the pencils, I can enjoy being creative, and random, and even breaking the rules and going over a line. This has taught me that there are, in fact, no rules! Think about it, where in the world is it written down that 'Thou shalt not go over the lines' or 'Thou shalt not put red next to purple'? By practicing mindfulness and noticing how your earlier trauma shows up in even quite silly activities such as colouring a picture or baking a cake, you can begin to change the rules and free yourself up to live life with more energy, creativity and joy. So, just to re-emphasise, colouring is not a cure for trauma or mental health crises and will not necessarily make you feel better, but it is a tool for developing mindfulness skills and may be helpful as part of a wider programme of self-development, self-care and self-healing.

Exercise 1

Let's practice a very simple mindfulness exercise to get present in this moment right here, right now. Most mindfulness trainings start by teaching you to focus on your breathing. It's a handy thing to practice on because it is, or at least should, always be with you! As Jon Kabat-Zinn says on his mindfulness app, referenced in Chapter 16, "if you're breathing right now then there's more right with you than wrong with you". The skill is to keep your mind on your breath for a few seconds, to a few minutes, building up to half an hour or more as you get more skilled. It sounds so simple, but let's just see what happens.

1. Find somewhere quiet and comfortable to sit.
2. Notice, if you are able to, the feeling of your body touching the chair and your feet on the floor. (Feel free to make any adaptations to the instructions to accommodate any disability issues you may have.)
3. Notice the feeling of your breath entering your nose.
4. Follow the sensations of your breath as it enters your lungs.
5. Notice the movements of your chest and abdomen as the breath fills you up.
6. Notice that moment as the in-breath stops, there is the briefest of pauses, and the breath turns around and begins to leave the body.
7. Notice the release as your body exhales.
8. Follow the sensations of the breath as it leaves through your nose or mouth.
9. Return to point 3 above and follow the next breath all the way in, and all the way out.
10. Repeat as often as you like.

It sounds so simple, but in fact, what you will notice is that your mind does not want to rest on the breath. It wants to wander around, looking for problems, looking for things to worry about, looking for new ideas. Buddhists refer to this as monkey-mind, where the mind wants to jump around and not be still. The mind has to be trained to be still and to focus to 'get in the zone'. At first you may only manage one in and out breath before your mind has wandered off. This is why we talk about mindfulness PRACTICE. We need a lot of practice to build up this skill, and breathing exercises are a perfect way of practicing. Don't beat yourself up if it feels too difficult; that is normal, and that is why we practice.

People who have experienced much trauma in their lives typically find these exercises far more challenging because their minds *really* do not want to be still, as it is in that stillness that memories and awful feelings can start to come to the surface. For this reason, it is important to take this at your own pace, slow and steady and not force it. If it is really unpleasant for you, stop, don't put pressure on yourself. I have heard of people going on silent meditation retreats to deal with difficulties in their life and being totally overwhelmed by the rush of things that come up when unprocessed trauma that has been held out of awareness for too long wells up in the silence and overflows, like a bottle of fizzy drink that has been shaken up and opened too quickly. If we think we may be full of shaken up fizzy drink, we need to take our lid off very slowly, in small increments, repeated over many attempts, to avoid it all spilling out and making a mess. Mindfulness practice needs to be done mindfully!

Emotional Openness

As we become more mindfully aware of the present moment and are more able to access this state moment by moment, we typically find our mind slows down, and we are more able to notice our emotions. This is vitally important as our emotions evolved as a way of helping us direct our actions in the interests of survival (Harris, 2019). Anger tells us when we have been wronged or are under threat and need to assert ourselves. Fear tells us when we are in danger and need to protect ourselves. Joy tells us when something is pleasurable, and we should do more of it. Shame tells us there is something wrong with us, and we need to change to fit in. Guilt tells us when we have wronged our community and need to make amends. As community is so vital to our survival, guilt and shame are very strong drivers of behaviour. All emotions are good emotions. They are there for very good survival reasons, and their original purpose was good. However, if we hold on to emotions, past their sell by date, they can become toxic.

An example of this is with shame. Let's imagine a little girl is sexually abused, let's call her Molly. Her abuser tells her it's a secret, and she must not tell otherwise something bad will happen to her mum. This is typical abuser behaviour. Molly knows that what happened was a bad thing and feels shame, which is very typical of children in such situations. She feels unable to tell, both because she is afraid of what will happen to her mum, as per the abuser's threats, and also because of the shame she feels. So, Molly hides the shame deep inside herself and keeps the secret. The shame festers inside her, perhaps for many decades. It makes her feel worthless in relationships. It stops her going for jobs or promotions. It makes her hide away rather than make friends and socialise. Molly perceives all this as failure, and new shame piles on top of the old shame.

Carolyn Spring, an author, abuse survivor and psychotherapist, discusses the role of shame in survivors of abuse (Spring, 2019). Spring describes how it is the connection between the survivor and a compassionate listener that breaks the shame. Being able to talk openly despite the shame in a relationship where there is no judgement, just acceptance and compassion, is the key to resolving shame. This is what we mean by emotional openness. First, opening up to oneself, recognising the emotions within and then being able to express those emotions, within a supportive relationship. That is what therapy should look like but can equally well happen between friends or family members, a close partner or spouse, or within social groups. My only words of caution here would be to go very carefully in opening up to others. Take your time and test them out with small truths and see how they respond. It is never a good idea to tell your whole story on first meeting someone new. This might overwhelm you, or them, and you need to see if they can be trusted with your truth before you share more fully.

Chapter Summary

- Mindfulness is about being aware of present moment reality, without judgement, with acceptance and compassion.
- There are many ways to develop mindfulness skills, and meditation is only one way.
- Traumatised people tend to find meditation difficult and can become easily overwhelmed when too much past trauma wells up in the silence of a meditation session.
- Physical activity can be a gentler way into mindfulness – a long swim, run, walk can give the mind time to settle.
- Creative pursuits such as art, craft, baking, gardening can have a similar effect.
- Breathing exercises and mindfulness apps are great if you can get along with them. Not everyone can and that is okay.
- None of these activities on its own is a cure for trauma, but mindfulness is a skill you will need to develop if you are to learn to cope better with what you have been through.
- Through developing mindfulness skills, you will gradually develop more emotional awareness.
- Cautious sharing of your emotional world in a supportive relationship can be enormously healing but should not be rushed.

13 Grounding/Getting Present

Obstacles to Getting Present

Being fully present is much more difficult if you have experienced a great deal of trauma, particularly if you tend to dissociate under pressure. Dissociation is a normal part of the trauma reaction (as discussed in Chapter 3) and can become a habitual way of dealing with strong emotions. People describe feelings of 'floatiness', 'spaciness', 'fogginess', 'disconnection', 'sleepiness' or things around them seeming strange, distorted or unreal. We all dissociate to a certain extent. Daydreaming is a form of dissociation. Highway amnesia – the feeling when you've taken a journey but cannot remember actually travelling parts of it – is a form of dissociation. We are often lost in our heads, holding conversations with imagined others, rehearsing what we will say to the boss or trying out different excuses for why we are home late. These are all examples of low-level dissociation.

Those of us who have experienced more extensive trauma and have used dissociation as a coping tactic might find that we spend large chunks of time 'zoned out'. We may be drifting through life with very little mindful awareness, and we may even think we have severe memory problems as we are so disconnected from what is going on that we can never remember where we put our keys, or whether we attended our child's parents' evening at school. People may get cross with us for never remembering conversations or for forgetting social engagements. We may find our concentration is poor, and we cannot even read a short article, never mind watch a whole movie.

At the more extreme end of the spectrum, we have those people who experienced such horrific trauma that they seem to have split off parts of their experience into dissociated parts of their self, which are usually kept well hidden from their own conscious awareness and out of sight of other people. In the more extreme cases, someone can be operating as a set of distinct but dissociated personalities where there will be a self that goes about everyday business, going to work and going to the doctor or the supermarket, but there will also be other parts of the self that sometimes take over that may represent strong emotions, traumatic memories or repressed parts of the self. To give an example, a person whose needs were never adequately met in childhood may have learnt to be very independent and can put on a good front to the world, as a capable, independent, hard-working person – that is their 'going about daily business part'. However, when faced with their needs being dismissed by a partner or friend, they may flip into a very needy, whiny, childlike person very different from their usual self. The more fragmented someone's personality is, the more disabling it can be as they may have no control over when their inner parts might start acting out, so they are seen as volatile, unpredictable or emotionally unstable. In some cases, we even see people having blackouts and seizures when memories or emotions are triggered, which is very alarming for all involved. Unfortunately, this is not well understood in medical circles, so is often dismissed as a 'behavioural problem' or 'attention seeking'.

As discussed in Chapter 5, there is a spectrum of dissociation from 'a bit daydreamy' to highly dissociative. 'A bit daydreamy' is about normal for most people whereas highly dissociative people may be diagnosed with a number of serious mental health conditions such as:

- Emotionally Unstable Personality Disorder
- Borderline Personality Disorder
- Dissociative Identity Disorder
- Post-Traumatic Stress Disorder
- Complex Post-Traumatic Stress Disorder
- Functional Neurological Disorder

If you find yourself at the less severe end of this spectrum, then learning to be present, mindful and grounded will be relatively easy. However, the more dissociative you are, the more difficult it becomes to learn these skills. Also, if much of your experience is held in dissociated memories and dissociated parts of yourself, then learning to be more grounded and less dissociated is going to lead to the whole of you becoming more aware of what you have been through, and this can be challenging.

The writings of Carolyn Spring are really excellent for understanding and managing severe dissociation (e.g. Spring 2019). Spring is a survivor of severe childhood abuse and has a diagnosis of dissociative identity disorder (DID). She describes her retreats into dissociation in the early stages of her therapy as a necessary coping strategy when her system was overwhelmed. Mental health professionals do not always know what to do in the face of such severe presentations and may take a punitive or highly critical approach. Spring tells of one therapist who told her to stop dissociating or else they could not help her when what she needed was someone to help her stay connected. Later, it was the compassionate, connected relationship with a different therapist that enabled her to become more coherent as a personality and be more in control of her need to dissociate. Spring tells us that simply telling someone to get present and stop dissociating will not work until the person has a good enough, connected relationship within which to begin the work.

What Is Grounding?

The skill of coming back to the present moment is called 'grounding' and can be a vital first step in managing any degree of dissociation and starting on a path towards greater mindfulness and healing of trauma. Quite literally, grounding is about coming back to earth from wherever your mind is wandering and coming back into yourself. I have a favourite set of exercises I use with people as a precursor to any trauma processing therapy which incorporates grounding, mindfulness and a little bit of imagination to create a sense of calm. I learnt this exercise when I attended a training workshop in the wake of the Manchester Arena terrorist bombing in 2017. Elan Shapiro, a highly respected

EMDR Consultant from Israel, was teaching a range of therapists and psychologists some skills and protocols for emergency trauma relief. He taught us his Four Elements Exercise as a quick way to help a person get grounded and present, ready for trauma processing (Shapiro, 2012). I have placed a handy guide to the Four Elements Exercise in the Appendix which you could screenshot onto your mobile phone for convenient access.

The Four Elements Exercise is a practical strategy that helps those dealing with the after-effects of trauma feel safe and stable. It involves focusing on the four separate elements (Earth, Air, Water and Fire) and using them as stepping stones to achieve a greater sense of grounding. When I use the Four Elements Exercise, I use it as an opportunity to teach the skills and also educate people on the processes involved in experiencing trauma symptoms and relieving them.

1. *Earth*

The first element is Earth, and this is where we ground ourselves and bring ourselves back to Earth, quite literally (if we can) by placing our feet on the floor and becoming aware of that pressure. As a double amputee, I cannot really do this, so I make myself aware of my body sitting in my chair, and the pressure points I can feel through my body touching the chair. We bring our awareness to the sensation of gravity holding us down, being anchored on the ground or in our chair. This begins to deal with the floaty, spacy feelings people have when dissociated. Just the act of pushing your feet into the floor brings your awareness to the present moment and starts to clear the fog. Then we begin to notice this moment, with all our senses, looking for five things we can see, four things we can hear, three things we can touch, two things we can taste and one thing we can smell. The order and the number of items do not matter, the point is that our efforts to use our senses to detect what is going on around us right now reinforce our attempt to be present and aware. We could also take a moment to notice the temperature of the room, the brightness of the light or any other sensations in the present moment.

2. *Air*

Once we are back in the room with our feet on the floor and our senses tuned back in, we turn our attention to the second element Air, by focusing on our breathing. I outlined a simple breathing exercise in Chapter 11 where I suggested following the in-breath and out-breath for a few breath cycles and building up from there. Concentrating on our breathing has a number of beneficial effects on us. When we are in a stressful situation and we go into fight/flight mode our breathing typically speeds up and becomes quite shallow, we hyperventilate and disrupt the balance of gasses in our bloodstream. This imbalance leads to unpleasant sensations such as light-headedness and tingling in our extremities. In a real emergency, that extra oxygen we breathe in through hyperventilon would be used up fuelling our muscles for the fight or flight, but in a panic attack, there is nowhere for that excess to go. Our brain takes this hyperventilation as a signal that there is something to panic about and escalates the stress response even further, becoming hyper-aroused, outside of our Window of Tolerance. Panic attacks then develop whereby we are hyped up ready for fight/flight, but there is nothing to fight or flee from. As we feel the panic, we notice our heart racing, our limbs shaking, our focus narrows, and we can feel dizzy, we begin to sweat, and our stomach churns. We can misinterpret these signals and think we are very sick, for example having a heart attack and dying, which only escalates the panic even further. Bringing our attention to our breath automatically starts to slow the panic process down, our breathing slows and deepens, and everything begins to settle. Getting our breathing under control is therefore one of the keys of calming the hyper-aroused nervous system, again bringing us back to earth and regulating our system.

There are many ways of regaining control of our breathing.

- First of all, just noticing that our breathing has changed is enough to start the process of re-regulating it.
- Second, we can make an effort to slow down and deepen our breathing, for example by taking longer, slower breaths all the

way down into our abdomen. Simply breathing out for a count of seven and in for a count of four for a few breaths helps to rebalance our blood gasses and regulate our nervous system.
- Third, there are a number of specific breathing exercises described in the appendix that can be used both as a meditation practice and as an emergency rescue strategy.

3. *Water*

The third element is Water, and here we use a simple skill to trick our nervous system out of fight/flight mode by using our imagination to get our mouth to water. As we have discussed at length earlier, when we are in fight/flight mode, our digestive system shuts down so that our energy and focus can be used most efficiently to save us from the threat. There's no point digesting our breakfast when we are about to be breakfast for the wolves! But once we have grounded ourselves and realised that there are no wolves, our body can still be caught in hyperarousal. So, then we use our imagination to switch our digestive system back on by imagining biting into a juicy lemon. This immediately makes our mouth water, which triggers a chain reaction from our mouth all the way down to our gut, telling our body we are now doing digestion, and we can stand down from the fight/flight response. Imagining biting into a lemon is, in my view, the single quickest way to stop a panic attack in its tracks.

4. *Fire*

Having used the Earth, Air and Water elements to bring ourselves out of our stress response, we can then use the fourth element, Fire, to light up our imagination and bring to mind whatever we need to help us through this moment. This might be our calm place, our happy place, our favourite activity, our best friend, someone we love, our spirit animal, our god or our favourite pet. It can be anything at all. We could imagine our favourite character from fiction, what would they do or say in this situation? We could imagine being in our favourite holiday destination and really feel the sights and sounds of the location. The power of our imagination is an often-untapped superpower for coping with life. Athletes, actors and musicians often use their imagination to visualise the perfect performance to great effect as a way of rehearsing when they cannot train or rehearse in real life.

There is a subtle difference between dissociation, which takes us over and disconnects us from what is important, and using our imagination deliberately to help us feel calm and connected in the present moment. Dissociation was a coping strategy during times of trauma, where we cut off automatically and zoned out from what was happening. This has become a habit that we are not in control of that leaves us feeling disconnected and adrift. Using our imagination to connect ourselves with helpful resources in a deliberate way is a more adaptive process because it is intentional, and we remain connected with the present moment, knowing that we are imagining a pleasant experience.

Calm Place Resource

Let's try firing up our imagination right now.

1) Bring to mind a wonderful place you have been, or can imagine being in, perhaps a beautiful beach, or a woodland scene, or somewhere you have seen on a travel show or in a movie.
2) Close your eyes and breath slowly and deeply as you imagine yourself there, what can you see? Take some time to look around and really bring the scene to life.
3) What can you hear? Listen carefully, are there birds singing, waves breaking, leaves rustling?
4) What can you smell? Take the time to notice the smells of nature, or food cooking or perfumes in the air.
5) What can you feel? Is there a breeze on your skin, sand between your toes, the sun on your face?
6) What can you taste? Is the air salty, or are you eating your favourite food in this lovely place?

7) Really take time with each sense to notice what is so wonderful about this place and as you enjoy the sensations, start to notice what is happening in your body as you relax into this calm, wonderful place in your imagination.
8) Notice as your breathing slows down and deepens. Notice the sense of calm in your mind and body. Notice your thoughts slowing down. Notice your muscles relaxing.
9) Now just spend a few moments enjoying this lovely experience.
10) Come back to it often and spend time here, just feeling calm and relaxed.

I have placed a quick guide to this exercise in the appendix so you can find it easily when you need it.

Practice, Practice, Practice

As with all the exercises I mention in this book, these things take practice, and you may not like them the first few times you do them. Ultimately it is up to you to find the ones you like best and go with them but do give them all plenty of tries before you abandon them. There are reasons why psychologists and therapists all use these exercises; it's because with practice they really do help people to move from struggling with trauma to coping with trauma. While I always teach the Four Elements Exercise in full, I recommend that people don't worry too much about getting it in the right order or doing the whole thing every time. It is, in fact, a bunch of helpful grounding and calming exercises that have been put together in a way that is easy to remember and incorporates many useful skills. Those skills can also be used separately in isolation from each other. Sometimes it is enough to simply push your feet into the floor to bring you back into the room, help you refocus, and you can get on with your day. Similarly, in a moment of panic, it may be enough to merely imagine biting into a lemon, to get your mouth watering and pull yourself out of panic mode. Equally, if you are trying to go to sleep and your mind is too busy, just bringing to mind your calm place, and settling into an exploration of the sights and sounds of that place, may be enough to quiet your mind and send you off to the land of nod. As with everything, there are no rules, just take what you can from these exercises and make them your own. One person I know took this set of exercises and rather than imagining biting into a lemon for the Water element, decided to carry around a tiny bottle of Tabasco sauce (pepper sauce) and literally took a drop onto their tongue whenever they needed to manage a panic. It certainly made their mouth water and took their mind off whatever was causing the panic! As I keep saying, there are no rules, 'do it your way', take what you can from me and make it your own!

Chapter Summary

- Dissociation is a normal part of trauma and gets in the way of our efforts to cope and heal.
- The more dissociative we are, the more difficult these skills are to learn; however, we can all learn to cope better, even from the worst of traumas.
- The Four Elements Exercise helps us to ground ourselves, regulate our breathing, calm our panic attacks and learn to relax.
- Our imagination is a superpower in learning to cope with trauma. Conjuring up a calm place, either from memory or simply making it up helps us to relax.
- Practice is crucial to our success with these exercises.

14 Dealing with Thoughts

Unhelpful Thoughts and Beliefs

In her book *Shattered Assumptions: Towards a New Psychology of Trauma*, Janoff-Bulman (1992) explains that when trauma happens it shatters our previously held assumptions that we are safe, other people are basically good and that the world is fundamentally safe. We assume that trauma happens elsewhere, to other people. When trauma then happens to us, we try to twist logic and come up with new, often unhelpful beliefs in order to make sense of it. For example, following a sexual assault, it is not unusual for a person to blame themselves. Rather than accept that awful things can happen, and we can be victims, it is somehow easier to believe that maybe it is our fault that we did something wrong that led to the assault. With this belief in mind, we then have the illusion that there is something we can do to prevent a future attack. Maybe we can dress differently, avoid certain places at certain times or drink less alcohol. This self-blame in relation to sexual assault is unfortunately reinforced by societal discourse and the actions of the criminal justice system which puts a lot of emphasis on how people can keep themselves safe, and less on how offenders might be encouraged to stop committing these crimes.

For people who grew up with neglect and abuse, or experienced prejudice and hatred from an early age, it is common to see very negative self-appraisals 'I'm worthless', 'I deserve bad things', 'I'm a bad person'. These are often then reinforced by further victimisation, for example within the education system. As discussed in Chapter 4 with the example of Jenny and Jake, Jake's inadequate upbringing leads to failure at school, which is met with punishment and exclusion, leading to further traumatisation and maladaptive coping, such as substance misuse and criminality. Jake is likely to believe that he deserves punishment, that he is a bad kid, that he is a failure and has let his hard-working mother down.

Combat veterans often struggle with negative self-beliefs when they have survived events that claimed the lives of their comrades. 'I should have died', 'it's my fault, I let my comrade down', 'I don't deserve to live', 'I don't deserve to enjoy my life now', 'my recovery would dishonour my fallen comrades'.

These negative self-beliefs drive behaviour which limits life and leads to anxiety and depression. Believing that you caused an adverse event leads to you avoiding anything which might cause a repetition of the event. For example, if you were assaulted in a nightclub, you may decide to avoid all nightclubs, not wanting to put yourself in the danger zone again, thus limiting your opportunities for enjoyment and socialising. If you believe you are a failure, you will avoid trying anything new, such as starting a course of study or applying for a new job, thus limiting your opportunities for financial security and independence. If you believe you let your comrades down and don't deserve a life now, you will struggle to re-engage in a satisfying civilian life. In these examples you may avoid further failure or further victimisation, but you also impose artificial restrictions on how satisfying life can be in the future.

Thought Challenging

One method that is taught in Cognitive Behavioural Therapy for dealing with unhelpful thoughts and beliefs is to challenge the thought by looking for evidence for and against it. To illustrate this with an example, let's imagine John has had a serious car accident. He was travelling on the motorway during rush hour, trying to get to an important meeting in another city. The weather was wet and misty, the traffic was heavy, and John was tired from working late on his laptop last night preparing for the meeting. As he listens to the radio and thinks through his pitch for the meeting a truck pulls out into the middle lane, forcing the car next to him to veer into his lane just ahead of him. John doesn't see all this unfold until the car clips his front wing, causing him to swerve out of control and be hit by the car behind him.

John is very upset and shaken, but thankfully not badly injured. He is checked out by the ambulance crew on the scene and told he is fit to go home. He arranges for his car to be recovered by his insurance company and his partner is able to come and pick him up. John is very disturbed by the accident and goes to see his doctor a few days later complaining of nightmares, angry outbursts, poor sleep and constant racing thoughts and images of the accident playing over in his mind. This is not untypical for someone who has been in such an accident. If John is well supported and well resourced, he should make a good recovery within a few weeks. However, John has always prided himself on being an excellent driver and having a clean driving record of no accidents and no speeding fines in 30 years of driving. His belief in himself as a good driver has been shattered by this experience. He ruminates endlessly on what he did wrong and how he could have let this happen. He was tired, he should have been focusing more. He had the radio on, he allowed himself to be distracted. He had not had sufficient rest; it is all his fault. He becomes fixed on these thoughts which maintains his disturbance about the accident and prevents him from resuming driving for longer than is really necessary.

If we get John to think about the accident and talk us through it, we might be able to challenge some of his unhelpful beliefs about it.

- Is it entirely his fault? He thinks so.
- Who pulled into the middle lane without looking? The truck driver did.
- Who swerved into John's lane? The other car driver did as he was avoiding the truck.
- Did the weather play a part? Yes, it did.
- Did the pressure from his boss to get this deal closed play a part? Yes, it did.

- Do accidents happen despite us taking every possible precaution? Yes, they do.
- If your partner was driving your car, would this accident be all their fault? No, of course not!

Challenging our unhelpful beliefs can be a really helpful way of shifting our perceptions and letting go of beliefs that are not serving us. For John, the belief that the accident was his fault causes him to delay getting back behind the wheel. The longer he avoids driving, the more anxious he becomes and the more he delays it. Not driving means he cannot return to work, so his life becomes increasingly restricted. The longer he delays his return to work, the more he blames himself for this new situation. The more he dwells on this, the harder it becomes to resume driving and overcome the natural anxiety anyone would have after such an accident.

Accepting Thoughts and Unhooking from Them

The risk with challenging our thoughts and trying to get rid of them is that we develop an obsession with them, becoming hooked on our negative self-belief. As we struggle to defeat our thoughts, we spend too much time caught up in them, and they become more and more powerful. The classic example used in therapy is telling someone not to think of a pink elephant, immediately all they can think of is pink elephants! In the example above, of John's car accident, it can happen that the more he tries to convince himself it was not entirely his fault, the more he becomes hooked on the idea that if only he had taken more precautions, he could have avoided it and, therefore, he is to blame.

The suggestion from ACT would be not to try to challenge or get rid of the belief, but rather to hold it lightly, and even playfully, in order to unhook ourselves from it. What this means is to notice our unhelpful thoughts, accept them and recognise them for what they are, just thoughts. Thoughts can be noticed, acknowledged, played with and let go gently. Russ Harris in his book *The Happiness Trap* (Harris, 2007) gives lots of examples of ways to play with and unhook from unhelpful thoughts. He suggests singing them to simple tunes, like Happy Birthday, saying them out loud in silly voices, or just repeating them until they get boring. He suggests imagining the thoughts are a radio playing in your head, Radio Doom and Gloom, he calls it and suggests just imagining turning the volume up and down on the radio to gain a sense of control. Accepting that we have unhelpful thoughts and beliefs and that we do not have to act on them or believe them can be very empowering.

In the example of John's car accident above, accepting that he is having the thought that the accident is his fault can help him to step back a little from actually believing it. It's just a thought, he can notice it and move on. Russ Harris recommends always thanking your mind for its intervention, 'Oh thanks, Mind, for making me think it's all my fault, that's really helpful – not!'. John can notice himself having that thought, thank his mind and then get on with the business of the day, which might involve driving somewhere. He might feel a little anxious but with practice, he will get back to his usual level of driving confidence. He might even choose to remind himself that he has had one serious accident in 30 years of driving, which is a pretty good record. Rather than dwelling on how much the accident was his fault, he is able to let go a little of the self-blame and concentrate on getting back to work and resuming his previous lifestyle.

Learning to Notice Our Thoughts Mindfully and Unhook

Learning to notice our thoughts mindfully without getting caught up in them and reinforcing them is a skill we can learn. It takes some practice but is very freeing once we have mastered it. The Leaves on the Stream exercise is a good way of developing and practicing the skill. Leaves on the Stream is a staple of mindfulness-based therapies and is taught as part of ACT. It is mentioned in *ACT Made Simple* (Harris,

2019), but I am not certain of its true origins, it may in fact predate modern therapy. There are many scripts for the exercise available online, and some audio versions you can listen to if needed; however, I have adapted my own version of the script from *ACT Made Simple* (2019) as follows:

1. Find a quiet and comfortable place to sit, where you will not be disturbed for a few minutes, maybe up to half an hour, maybe longer. The duration of the exercise is up to you.
2. Imagine you are sitting beside a river or a stream with the water flowing gently past, not a raging torrent, and not still waters, something gentle, but moving.
3. Picture your surroundings, maybe you are sitting on a comfortable log beside the river's edge, maybe there are trees overhanging the water, dropping the occasional leaf onto the surface of the water, maybe you can hear birdsong or the rustling of the wind in the trees. Make the scene your own and embellish it however you like.
4. Imagine yourself sitting here, enjoying a few moments of peace and tranquillity away from the usual hassles of daily life.
5. Always, when we start to relax and take a break like this, our mind starts to get busy, that's normal, don't try to fight it, in fact, do the opposite, accept it and just notice each thought as it pops into your mind.
6. As you notice each thought, imagine yourself placing it on a leaf on the surface of the river and watch as it either hangs around or floats away in its own good time.
7. It matters not whether these are good thoughts, bad thoughts or somewhere in the middle thoughts, they are just thoughts and can be placed on a leaf to do as they wish.
8. Try not to force anything, try to just notice. Don't try to push the thoughts away, place them on a leaf and just be curious.
9. If there are no thoughts, just notice that and watch the river flowing by while you listen to the sounds of nature all around. If

your mind is a human mind, you can be sure it will start up with the random thoughts again very soon.
10. Spend as long as you like on this exercise and practice it regularly.

What the Leaves on the Stream exercise teaches us is that we don't need to analyse every thought we have, and we certainly don't need to believe every thought either. I tend to have a very busy mind that is hard to shut off at times. When I am stressed, I notice old unhelpful beliefs tend to creep back into my thought process. For example, if I have been challenged by another professional on a piece of work, my immediate thoughts would be 'I've got it wrong', 'I've screwed up', 'How can I put this right?', and these thoughts might play on my mind late at night when I should be sleeping. I now recognise that these thoughts have their origins in early criticism and emotional abuse I received growing up. I can now recognise when this is happening and use mindfulness techniques to unhook myself from the thoughts and let them go. Having practiced the Leaves on the Stream exercise many times, I can bring it to mind very easily and put all those unhelpful thoughts onto the leaves and watch them float away. Or I can simply say to myself, 'Oh it's that old story, I'm a failure, I'm useless, thanks Mind, but I don't need to think about that right now as I want to go to sleep'. I can then turn my attention to how tired my body feels, how comfortable my bed is, how heavy my eyelids are and maybe bring to mind a calm place with soothing sounds and images. By unhooking from the unhelpful thought stream and coming back to present moment awareness, I am much more able nowadays to get to sleep even when I have had a stressful experience that would, in the past, have kept me awake for hours.

The Emotional Impact of Thoughts

One important reason for learning to manage our difficult thoughts is the emotional impact they have on us. Imagine you are constantly having the unhelpful thought, 'I'm worthless'. How is that going to make you feel? Of course, it will make you *feel* worthless and full of shame, it will adversely impact your self-esteem and cause low mood. Over time, you will become depressed, lose motivation and give up on any aspirations you once had. When we are depressed, often we don't really understand why we are depressed, we just are. Spending time on exercises such as Leaves on the Stream can help us gain insight into our emotional state as well as our thoughts. If we are trudging through life full of unkind thoughts about ourselves, feeling miserable and dwelling in the awfulness of it all, it is very difficult to start making changes for the better. This growing awareness of our inner world of thoughts and feelings that comes from mindfulness exercises such as Leaves on the Stream can then help us to make more mindful choices about what we do next.

Self-Compassion

The awareness that we gain through these exercises begins to create changes in us without us necessarily having to put in much effort. Simply being able to notice a self-critical thought and the shame that comes with it might lead you to say to yourself, 'Gosh, that was such an unkind thought, I'm really not that bad, am I?' Once you start noticing how unkind you are to yourself, it becomes much easier to see why you feel so down so much of the time, and you may start to feel greater warmth and compassion for yourself. You might even start responding to your inner dialogue with more kindness and compassion. This is not a given, and the more trauma you have experienced the more work may be required to build self-compassion. Again, it's a matter of how well resourced you are from childhood and how well you are able to respond to yourself with compassion and loving kindness. You may be the world's most compassionate person when it comes to other people's struggles, but it is how you relate to yourself that really impacts how you feel day to day. People who work hard to bring care and kindness to others, whilst neglecting their own need for compassion, tend to burn out so it is very important that we notice this in ourselves and make time to work on our self-compassion skills. The old adages about putting your own oxygen mask on before helping others or not being

Dealing with Thoughts

able to feed others from an empty cup are very relevant here. You have to learn to apply at least the same level of compassion to yourself as you would to another person.

A practice you can use to develop greater self-compassion uses your imagination to create your own inner cheerleader, nurturer and supporter figure. We use this type of imagined resource figure a lot in EMDR therapy, but it is also used in Compassion Focused Therapy and more than likely in many other forms of therapy. Some people find it harder than others to use their imagination to conjure something from nothing, if that is the case for you, then use someone or something more real from your own experience rather than something completely imagined.

1. Take a few moments to settle your mind in a quiet, comfortable place. Slow your breathing and relax your body as best you can.
2. Try to bring to mind a person or a creature from real life, from fiction, from a movie or from your own imagination who is kind, caring and compassionate.
3. Think what they would look like. How big are they? How are they dressed? How do they look at you?
4. Notice how they move. Are they dancing alongside you? Are they floating above you? Are they following you closely?
5. Notice what they say. Are they encouraging you? Are they using supportive words and facial expressions? Are they telling you not to worry if you make mistakes?
6. Really take some time to build your character or to recall them if they are from real life, noticing all the aspects of how they look, move and communicate with you.
7. Ensure that this character is unfailingly supportive and kind, never critical or judgemental.
8. Bring this character to mind every time you find yourself struggling or in need of encouragement. Imagine them cheering you on, congratulating you and consoling you when things don't go so well.

When I first came across this exercise in Paul Gilbert's *The Compassionate Mind* (Gilbert, 1992), I immediately recalled an image from my very young childhood where I had thought I had seen a white witch at the window. I don't know to this day what I had actually seen, maybe just a figment of a childish imagination. However, as soon as I read through this exercise, that image came to mind, and she has become my inner cheerleader ever since. She's sitting on the sofa in my office right now with her funny pointy white hat and flowing white gown, telling me that although writing a book is hard, it is valuable work and will be so worthwhile when it is done. I'm trying very hard to believe her.

Chapter Summary

- Trauma instils in us all sorts of unhelpful beliefs which pop into our minds constantly causing us to feel low and anxious.
- Often our unhelpful beliefs are a way to feel more in control – if it was my fault then maybe I can do things differently to stop it from happening again.
- These unhelpful beliefs may have seemed helpful to us at one time, but they hold us back and stop us from fulfilling our aspirations.
- We can try to challenge our unhelpful thoughts by looking for evidence, but we must not get so involved in them that we become hooked onto them.
- We can learn to unhook ourselves from unhelpful thoughts through mindfulness exercises such as the Leaves on the Stream.
- Mindfulness practices help us to recognise the link between thoughts and emotions and help us to become much more aware of our inner world.
- A natural and very necessary progression from mindfulness practice is the development of self-compassion.

15 Valued Living and Thriving

Valued Living

In ACT, we believe the key to living a satisfying life is to accept what we can't change, to connect with our values and live according to them. Values can be anything that makes life meaningful for you. Going back to the idea of the A-C-E pie chart in Chapter 8, we need to be living our lives in the domains of Achievement – Enjoyment – Connection. We can break each of these domains down into smaller sub-domains, so Achievement might include work, study, volunteering, personal challenges and so on. Enjoyment might include hobbies, play, reading for fun. Connection might include community activities, socialising, family activities, friendship. There are no rules here, it's your life, you fill it with what you want. It is worth making sure though that you don't over-attend to one area and neglect the others. Putting all your attention on success at work might leave you with little social connection and may threaten any relationships in your life. The old adage that nobody on their deathbed ever says they wish they had spent more time at the office applies here.

Importantly, there is not a set of correct values to have, it's not a case of having the right or wrong values. Often when I try to discuss values with clients, they begin by thinking about morality and what makes a person objectively good. That is not the sort of values we are talking about here. We are talking about what makes life feel meaningful and worthwhile *for you*. In other words what do *you* value? What made life feel good to Genghis Khan or Adolf Hitler will look very different from what made life feel good to the Buddha or Mahatma Gandhi, and there are infinite possibilities between these vastly different positions. While one person may value wealth, power and world domination, others may value kindness, service and care. The important thing is to consider what matters most to you.

Prior to the pandemic that began in early 2020, when I worked in an office and saw people in person for therapy, I would use a set of values cards to help people narrow down their values to the most important few. Sorting these cards is a way to help someone think about their values and identify which ones are really important to them. Seeing all the options helps to reinforce the idea that there is no right or wrong here, your values are your values. Anyone else can choose their own from the deck of cards. Each card has just one word as follows, see Table 15.1:

POWER	SERVICE	KINDNESS	WEALTH	HEALTH	CHALLENGE
CURIOSITY	LEARNING	LEADERSHIP	FRIENDSHIP	CHARITY	FAMILY
FUN	FULFILMENT	TRUST	COMPASSION	LOVE	HONESTY
SUPPORT	FAIRNESS	INTEGRITY	LOYALTY	ACHIEVEMENT	ENCOURAGE-MENT
HAPPINESS	JOY	BEAUTY	STRUCTURE	ORDER	SELF RESPECT
RESPECT	INNER PEACE	WINNING	PATIENCE	SAFETY	SECURITY
SPIRITUALTY	HOPE	INNER STRENGTH	PASSION	WISDOM	CONSISTENCY
NATURE	NURTURE	PEACE	GRATITUDE	COURAGE	ADVENTURE
CREATIVITY	HOME	INDEPENDENCE	CONNEC-TION	DIGNITY	SENSUALITY
ACCEPT-ANCE	FREEDOM	ADVENTURE	RISK	CARING	EQUALITY

TABLE 15.1 Values

There is also an app for mobile devices called ACT Coach, which was developed for military veterans in the USA, details of the app can be found in Chapter 16. ACT Coach helps you with all the skills we are discussing here, including helping you to narrow down your values and think about the small committed actions you could take each day in the service of those values. By narrowing these values down to the five or six most strongly resonant ones, we can start to think about how we live each of those values in daily life. This can take the form of small steps, repeated often, or major leaps in a new direction, or anything in between. One of my most strongly held values is around learning. I have always been a sponge for new knowledge and skills and am constantly on the search for new ideas. This quest extends to sharing my learning with others and as I have become more skilled and accredited in my field of expertise, I have increasingly dedicated time to developing and training others in the field too. I get a real buzz from supervising and training others, but there was a time when my lack of self-confidence would have precluded me from even considering this. 30-year-old-me would be truly shocked to see 55-year-old-me delivering group supervision to experienced psychologists. The reason being that 30-year-old-me still had a lot of work to do on herself to identify and connect with her values and to let go of some of the barriers that held her back from living in tune with those values.

Barriers to Valued Living

Some people really struggle to let go of the idea that there are right and wrong choices to be made here, particularly if they have a people-pleasing tendency. However, if you are living your life according to someone else's values out of fear of offending others, then life will simply not be as satisfying to you as it would be if you were living more in tune with your values. Culture can play a part in pushing people to live out of kilter with their values. Historically, women in white western societies were brought up to prioritise marriage and having children, to be self-sacrificing in the interests of family and not to prioritise their own career aspirations. Feminist backlash against traditional roles for women in the 1960s and 1970s in the United States and United Kingdom, in particular, led to my generation of women believing we can 'have it all' in terms of career and family. Unfortunately, society has not entirely let go of the idea that women remain responsible for the home and family and work often has been simply another thing we have been expected to do. I hear from many very successful middle-aged professional businesswomen in therapy that they are struggling to hold everything together as they feel they were sold a lie. There very much needs to be balance and fairness if everyone is to be able to live a valued life.

When people have experienced significant trauma in their lives and survival has been the only priority, they may never have had the opportunity to stop and wonder what they really want. Again, it goes back to Maslow's hierarchy (see Chapter 8). You must get the bottom layers of safety and stability in place before you can start assessing what would make for a truly meaningful life. People in deep struggle tend not to have as many choices open to them. Remember Jenny in Chapter 4 coming from a deprived background in care, pregnant before she completed school and trying to bring up her child in poor socio-economic conditions? She needs a great deal of support if she is ever to achieve her true potential and live a fully satisfying life. As a young single mum with no support, she has very few options other than to engage in a constant hustle for basic survival. With the right support though, she may be able to complete her education, gain meaningful employment and achieve a more stable life for herself and her child. Only then can she really think about what else she wants and needs beyond that.

Society has a vital part to play in supporting people to make the choices that will enable them to recover from trauma and live well. Women need flexibility in the workplace and affordable childcare. Men need to step up and support women with the domestic load. People who are held back by early deprivation, abuse and neglect need social services and financial support to enable them to build the foundations of a good life. Adequate benefits need to be available that allow young people leaving the care system or escaping from abusive homes to be able to complete their education and live safely away from drugs and gangs so that they can build a meaningful and worthwhile life. Inequalities around race, ethnicity, disability, age, gender, sexuality, all need to be addressed at a societal and institutional level. Until structural inequality is addressed, it remains difficult for less privileged people to really make the choices that will add value into their lives and as a result add value back into society.

Putting Values into Practice

We need to be able to get a little bit mindful if we are to connect with our values. We need to let go of judgement, there are no 'right' values in this context. We need to create a little time and space to just notice what matters to us. The values table above is also in the appendix and you can copy it and cut it up into individual cards. Once you have made a bit of time and space for yourself and focused your mind on the task, the first step is to divide the cards into two piles – 'matters to me' and 'doesn't matter to me'. The next step is to take the 'matters to me' pile and repeat the exercise just with those cards. The idea is that you reduce the pile by about half each time until you get down to about a maximum of six cards. These are your core values right now. Notice them and think about how you are living each of those values in your life today. Alternatively, you can identify your key values through the ACT Coach app as discussed above.

I have worked with people who have realised through this exercise that they were completely neglecting a core value. For example, the self-employed businessperson who realised they had completely neglected their need to travel as they have been so absorbed in the work and family hustle. The person who realised that their high-earning finance role didn't adequately meet their value of helping others. The mum who valued study but had never pursued that path because children came along, and she had to prioritise their needs. Getting a sense of what would make life more meaningful helps us to then make choices, moment by moment, towards a more satisfying life.

Post-Traumatic Growth

When people experience traumatic events, it creates a period of adjustment and reflection. If there are physical or psychological injuries, a person needs to take time to process what has happened and to heal as best they can. In my case, when I had begun to recover from meningitis and septicaemia at age 19, I had to adjust to using a wheelchair and being seen as a disabled person. Such events really do make you stop and think. I nearly died back there, and what had I done with my life? What did I want going forward? If I was going to survive, what sort of life did I want? These were very big questions at such a young age. I do believe though that the questions I asked of myself during that period of my life set me on a path towards a paralympic basketball career and becoming a clinical psychologist. For me, those outcomes represented personal growth far beyond anything that my path prior to the illness seemed to be leading towards.

During my clinical psychology doctoral training, I wrote my thesis on the topic of Post-Traumatic Growth. It was a topic I identified strongly with, and it seemed under-researched at the time. It is a potentially controversial topic as the study of it almost creates an expectation that this should be the goal. If personal growth through trauma is the goal, what if you don't experience any growth? Have you failed at being a trauma survivor? People's outcomes after trauma depend on many factors – what internal and external resources they had prior to the trauma, societal privilege, extent of injuries incurred, support available and many more. I have mentioned before that luck is a huge factor in how trauma and disability impacted me and how I was able to recover and thrive in its wake. Had I not had educational and social advantages, had I not met the right people at the right time, had I not been able to claim certain benefits, my post-traumatic pathway might have looked very different. Whilst acknowledging that recovery and personal growth rely on many factors that may be out of your control, I could not ignore this area of research in a book about coping with trauma.

The study of post-traumatic growth began in the early 1990s following two shipping disasters involving significant loss of civilian life. In March 1987, the *Herald of Free Enterprise* passenger ferry sank just outside of the Belgian port of Zeebrugge en route to Dover in Kent, then in October 1988, a cruise ship, the *Jupiter*, was sunk in an accident off the coast of Greece carrying a party of 400 British schoolchildren and their teachers. Many of the survivors of both of these events were later treated for post-traumatic stress disorder. However, in treating the traumatised survivors, researchers also discovered positive changes in outlook following the trauma and began to research that (Joseph, Williams & Yule, 1993). Further research in the United States in the 1990s and early 2000s built on this idea that trauma can lead to positive outcomes beyond what may have been expected had the trauma not occurred. Tedeschi and Calhoun (2004) identified five domains of growth arising out of the struggle to process traumatic events, namely:

- Improved relationships
- Sense of new possibilities in life
- Increased appreciation of life
- Sense of personal strength
- Spiritual development

My own research in 2004–2006 looked specifically at people who had experienced disabling illnesses or injuries (Waft, 2006). I interviewed a self-selected sample of people who identified with the theme of post-traumatic growth to try to understand more about what the process was that had taken these people from surviving to thriving. I interviewed a disability rights activist, an artist, a solicitor, a student, an adaptive technology designer and a retired charity worker. Reviewing my findings from a position many years later, I would sum it up as follows:

1. First, people had to really acknowledge and take stock of what had happened to them, creating a distance between themselves and their trauma with its ensuing struggles. So, this meant seeing the trauma and the struggles as separate from the self and locating the trauma in history – 'I am not my trauma' and 'my trauma is then, not now'. This allowed them to acknowledge the reality of the trauma without being weighed down by it in the present.
2. Second, people really had to wrestle with balancing positives and negatives in their situation, acknowledging the struggle, but not missing the rays of sunlight in between. This might take the form

of losing one career, whilst appreciating having more time with family or developing a newer, more fulfilling career in a different field.
3. Third, people took a lot of effort over reviewing their identity, their values and what really mattered to them. For example, nearly dying made people question how much time they had spent at the office chasing material wealth versus how much time they had spent on other pursuits. Most felt that their lives were richer for having resolved these dilemmas according to their values.
4. Finally, people talked at length about making meaning from their experiences, and this took many forms. There were themes about seeking a new purpose, taking on new roles, taking up new challenges. This included a sense of 'giving back' in some way, fundraising for causes, working in disability rights advocacy or even taking a whole new career path to help others.

I very much identify with the themes that came out in my research. It was not an overnight process for myself or any of my research participants. Some were reflecting on this many years or even decades after their original trauma. My big traumatic illness was back in 1986, and it has been a bumpy road at times from then to now. Post-traumatic growth does not come about through denial of the struggle or putting a happy face on it. It comes about through embracing the challenges, sitting with the messy feelings and making hard choices to move forward. One of my research participants had such a hard struggle with the legal process following their accident, they retrained in the law and became a lecturer in law so that they could impact future generations of legal trainees. This involved being rightfully angry and channelling that into positive action and very hard work over many years. For me, it was similar, a sense of there being a lack of support after my illness left me wondering what support there ought to have been and this led me, in a roundabout way, into studying psychology and ultimately specialising in trauma therapy work.

When we talk about values, it is important not to get into comparisons or assume that everyone should have the same values as you. Equally, post-traumatic growth might look very different from one person to another. I mentioned toxic positivity in Chapter 10, and I think there is a danger of getting into a similar thing with post-traumatic growth. How many times do we read about someone trekking across the Arctic, up a mountain or across a desert wilderness after surviving cancer, losing a limb or being in some other way affected by trauma? It is a theme beloved by the mainstream western media. A tragic story about a dreadful event, followed by the inspirational recovery and amazing feat of endurance. The triumph over tragedy narrative is popular and can be very damaging to people when they are just trying to survive and do their best.

Chapter Summary

- Values are about living our lives in the most fulfilling way for us.
- There is no right or wrong set of values.
- Society and culture have a huge impact on the extent to which any individual can live according to their values.
- When we reflect on our values, we can make decisions about our life that feel more congruent with who we are.
- Reflecting on our values and redirecting our life following trauma can lead to post-traumatic growth, the move from surviving to thriving.
- Post-traumatic growth can lead to improvements in all areas of our lives but is not necessarily a goal or expectation for everyone.

16 Conclusions and Further Help

Understanding Trauma

Trauma has been an important area of study for well over a hundred years, from Freud and Charcot in the late 1800s through Judith Herman in the 1990s, to our present understandings informed by neuroscience and brain imaging. I was drawn to study the psychology of trauma and work with trauma survivors following my own experiences of childhood adversity and medical trauma in early adulthood. In this book I wanted to bring together my knowledge of the theory of trauma as we now understand it with my own personal journey of healing and coping with trauma.

Understanding some of the theory of trauma is vitally important in helping to address the complex ways that we respond to these overwhelming experiences. Often people come into therapy saying they are 'going mad' or 'losing their mind'. Others are beating themselves up for not being able to simply stop a coping strategy that has got out of hand, such as drinking or self-harming. Once we understand the theory and can see what is happening in our minds and our bodies, our attempts to cope make a lot more sense, and we can begin the task of finding new more helpful ways to cope.

I have described different types of trauma from simple, single incident traumas in adulthood, through to the more complex, developmental traumas caused by neglect, abuse and poor attachments in childhood. I have described little-t traumas and big-T traumas. I have described the way trauma impacts multiple generations of families and communities, even societies on a global scale. When unresolved trauma causes people to act in ways that harm others there is an urgent need for psychologically informed interventions to break the cycle of harm.

Conclusions and Further Help

I have explored the impact trauma has on our physical and mental wellbeing, drawing on the ACE studies from the early 1990s. I have looked at how the multifaceted nature of our lives leads to different outcomes for different people. I have considered how our diverse characteristics can either lessen or worsen our experience of trauma, noting for example how my educated, white British status, and the luck of having access to a functioning National Health Service right when I needed it, helped ensure I was not only able to survive, but to thrive following my brush with meningitis. How different might this have been had I had racism, low educational attainment or other social disadvantages to deal with as well? So many physical and mental health conditions seem to have their roots in trauma. Trauma overwhelms our ability to cope in the moment and if left unresolved has far reaching consequences for our future well-being.

I have expanded on the impact of trauma to include the very complex presentations we see in clinical practice, where early trauma has caused severe dissociation and fragmentation of the sense of self. These presentations have long been a topic of study among psychologists and therapists but remain somewhat controversial. Dissociation, fragmentation and the risks that go with these more severe trauma presentations need special attention and may not be resolved through a self-help book alone. I hope that this book at least gives you a starting point for your own healing journey.

Modern neuroscience has helped us to understand a great deal about how trauma impacts the brain. It is not an easily accessible area of study for many of us and I have simplified my understanding of it as best I can for the lay reader. Neuroimaging has enabled scientists to see inside living brains as they process events and information, giving live data on key brain systems involved in processing traumatic events. Theories such as the Triune Brain Theory help to simplify some of this complex science so that we can understand what happens when we face a traumatic event, and when we later try to process that. Understanding that our brains have evolved to act instinctively in moments of severe threat can help us to let go of self blame and guilt for our actions. Knowing that the ways we are struggling now were part of our best attempts at coping then can help us feel less ashamed of our struggles and more compassionate towards ourselves. For neurodivergent people this is even more important to recognise as trauma impacts the neurodivergent brain more severely and neurodivergent people face more trauma generally.

Trauma does not only impact the human mind, but also the body. We recognise that the body often holds an imprint of a psychological trauma, such as in the case of Irritable Bowel Syndrome. We see many chronic pain conditions and medically unexplained illnesses which may have their roots in psychological trauma. Whether there is a trauma at the heart of a symptom we may never know, but nonetheless, I believe the strategies offered in this book may go some way to relieving the experience of living with that symptom. There are some schools of psychotherapy that focus entirely on the bodily experience to relieve symptoms of trauma.

The Healing Journey

I use the analogy of peeling an onion to describe how trauma therapy typically goes. First we have to gently deal with the tough outer skin, by which I mean the resistance and unhelpful coping strategies that get in the way of us living our best life. We do this by developing new skills such as mindfulness, grounding and gaining balance between the 3 areas of achievement, enjoyment and connection with others. Then we process the onion ready for cooking, by which I mean we confront the trauma and process it, putting it firmly in the past. Then we look at how to make a dish worth eating, or a life worth living, focusing on what makes life meaningful for us and taking brave little steps towards a rewarding future.

The first stage involves recognising that what were helpful coping strategies at the time of the trauma, may have become dysfunctional behaviours over time that no longer serve us so well. We need to learn to use coping strategies in a healthy mindful way, whilst still confronting our difficult feeling and memories. In order to do this we need to build up our resources, widen our Window of Tolerance and gain some mastery over our vagus nerve. All of this is achieved using mindful activity, learning to ground ourselves, learning to use our breath to regulate ourselves and using imagined resources where possible to calm ourselves. All of this is again more difficult for neurodivergent people, so more support and specialist skill may be needed at all stages of the process. Having the right people around us, having knowledge of trauma and having the right skills are the crucial ingredients to coping with trauma.

Acceptance and Commitment Therapy (ACT)

I draw heavily on ACT in my work with traumatised people and in this book. ACT has been around since the 1990s and draws heavily on older philosophies from the far east as well as very western ideas from cognitive and behavioural therapies. Within ACT we are encouraged to be mindfully present with whatever is happening in this moment, right here right now, with acceptance, compassion and non-judgement. From this stance we learn to confront our present reality with openness, letting go of avoidance. We learn to really feel whatever is there, however painful, and to respond with compassion.

Some people may use meditation as a way to access mindfulness and there are many apps available on your mobile device to help you practice this. I have listed a few of these apps later in this chapter. Other ways of accessing mindfulness are through physical exercise (yoga, running, swimming are all good examples); through creating art or craft; through music, either listening to music, or playing an instrument; through other creative pursuits such as cooking or baking; through connecting with nature (open water swimming, hiking, gardening, walking the dog). As you spend more time mindfully attending to such activities, you will gradually open up to your inner emotional experience. Cautious sharing of that within supportive relationships can help to begin processing the difficult feelings and memories.

Depending where you are starting from on the spectrum of complexity (simple trauma to very severe complex trauma) you will need to spend more or less time on learning to ground yourself and become aware of the present moment. I offer the Four Elements Exercise as a way for anyone to start building these skills. The key to success with this is practice, practice and more practice. There are no shortcuts here.

As we become more aware of our present moment, we notice the content of our thoughts more clearly and this can be eye opening! All too often, trauma leaves us with unhelpful beliefs about ourselves, other people and the world which cause unhelpful thoughts to cascade endlessly through our minds. We can try to challenge our unhelpful thoughts and beliefs. If we notice the thought 'I'm unworthy' we could challenge that and tell ourselves 'I am worthy', but unfortunately that rarely sticks for long. In ACT, we learn to simply notice the thought and any emotions that go with it, then thank our mind and move on to something more useful. When we stop getting into a struggle with these thoughts and feelings, we notice they become less intrusive and less persistent. As we become more skilled at simply noticing in this way, we are also naturally more likely to become less critical of ourselves and more compassionate.

The final part of the puzzle is to connect with our values and start taking those tiny steps towards our valued future. This refers to whatever makes life meaningful to you, no-one else, just you. There are no right or wrong values to hold. Reflecting on our values following a traumatic event, or even following a lifetime of trauma, can lead to us making changes that allow us not only to survive, but often to thrive. Post traumatic growth can then be an unexpected outcome of trauma, although it is not required.

Seeking Further Help and Support

For some people, a traumatic event can lead to or exacerbate mental health difficulties, such as post-traumatic stress disorder (PTSD), anxiety disorders or depression. Whilst you may experience many of the symptoms below in the immediate aftermath of your traumatic event, they should resolve naturally within a few weeks to a few months in approximately 70% of cases. However, there may be cause for concern if these persist.

Symptoms of PTSD:
1. **'Intrusion Symptoms'** such as unwanted thoughts, images, emotions and body sensations. This would include flashbacks, where a person vividly re-experiences aspects of the disturbing event as if it was actually happening again, and nightmares.
2. **'Avoidance Symptoms'** such as avoiding thoughts and feelings about the disturbing event by using distraction techniques, using alcohol or drugs, keeping extremely busy, refusing to talk about the disturbing event and avoiding external reminders of the disturbing event such as certain people, places and situations.
3. **'Mood and Cognition Symptoms'** such as anxiety, low mood, negative beliefs about the self and strong emotions such as fear, horror, anger, guilt or shame.
4. **'Hyperarousal Symptoms'** such as irritability, angry outbursts, jumpiness, poor sleep, inability to relax and hyper-vigilance (being on high alert).

Symptoms of Depression:
1. Feeling down or hopeless
2. Little interest or pleasure in things you usually enjoy
3. Feeling bad about yourself
4. Feeling irritable
5. Feeling tired, lacking energy
6. Difficulty concentrating
7. Difficulty sleeping, or wanting to sleep all the time
8. Loss of appetite or overeating
9. Thoughts of suicide or of not wanting to be around

Symptoms of Anxiety:

1. Feeling nervous or anxious
2. Difficulty relaxing
3. Ongoing worrying thoughts
4. Worrying about lots of different things
5. Fearing the worst
6. Feeling irritable
7. Feeling restless or agitated

If you find you are experiencing several of these symptoms persistently, you should seek further help. Please do not feel you need to try to cope on your own. There is help available. It is also important that you tell a family member or friend how you are feeling so that they can help you to access the support you need and hopefully be available as an additional source of support.

Where to Seek Further Support

1. If you are being treated for physical illness or injuries in the aftermath of your traumatic event, your medical team may have access to psychological therapies with a clinical, counselling or health psychologist as part of the service they offer, so it is worth asking there as a first step. These are highly trained and regulated Practitioner Psychologists who are trained to work with people struggling with the emotional impact of physical health problems, illness and disability.
2. In the UK, your GP (Primary Care Physician) will have the best knowledge of what general mental health support is available in your area. Whilst it can often be difficult to get an appointment, and there may be long waiting lists, it is really important that you reach out in relation to mental health difficulties.
3. Again, in the UK, you should be able to self-refer to your local NHS Talking Therapies (previously known as Improving Access to Psychological Therapies (IAPT) service). These services offer

short-term counselling and therapies to people experiencing common mental health difficulties. More information can be found on the NHS website.
4. If you wish to see a psychologist privately, it is important to ensure you see someone who is highly trained and regulated. In the UK, the term 'psychologist' is not a protected title. Therefore, you should seek someone who is registered with the Health & Care Professions Council (HCPC). Anyone calling themselves a clinical, health, forensic or counselling psychologist in the UK should be registered with HCPC. You can check the register on the HCPC website. For more on finding a clinical psychologist, the Association of Clinical Psychologists UK (ACP-UK) has a useful guide on its website.

If You Are at Risk to Yourself

Some people who have been through traumatic events may have thoughts of self-harm and suicide, and these thoughts may become more frequent and concerning over time. As stated above, thoughts of suicide or not wanting to be around can be an indication of depression. If you notice **any of the below** symptoms, then you should seek immediate help:

- Being preoccupied with thoughts of death or dying,
- Making a plan of how you would end your life,
- Taking steps to say goodbye to loved ones,
- Acquiring things to follow through with your plan,
- Writing a suicide note.

Where to Seek Further Crisis Support

1. It is important to let your GP know about any of these symptoms. Ask for an urgent appointment.
2. If you live in England, you can access the NHS Urgent Mental Health helpline via the NHS website.

3. The Samaritans are trained to support people who are feeling suicidal. You can call them for free at any time on 116 123. There are also other ways to get in touch with the Samaritans on their website.
4. If you are concerned that you are at high or immediate risk of suicide, then you should go to the Accident & Emergency Department at your local hospital. There will be a psychiatric liaison team on duty who will be able to assess you and work with you to develop an immediate plan to support you.

Therapies for Resolving Trauma

In the UK all medical and mental health treatment is overseen by the National Institute for Health and Care Excellence (NICE). NICE evaluates the research and makes recommendations as to what treatments are considered safe and effective for all conditions. The NICE Guidelines for the treatment of PTSD were reviewed and updated in 2018 (NICE 2018). NICE recommends both trauma-focused Cognitive Behavioural Therapy (TF-CBT) and Eye Movement Desensitisation and Reprocessing (EMDR) Therapy for the treatment of PTSD.

At the time of writing, both TF-CBT and EMDR are well supported by robust research evidence and are internationally recognised as effective trauma treatments. Other forms of therapy such as Acceptance and Commitment Therapy have a developing evidence base in the treatment of trauma. It is important that any therapy you choose has been shown to work with the sort of difficulties traumatised individuals face. There are many unvalidated, untested therapies being used by people with limited training and knowledge. In the field of trauma and mental health, there are severe risks that can arise if untrained individuals attempt to treat people without the necessary awareness and knowledge. For example, if trauma therapy is taken too fast, without the necessary stabilisation skills in place, people can become overwhelmed with trauma memories and may dissociate and/

or become suicidal. It is therefore necessary to find a practitioner with the appropriate background in trauma and mental health, such as a Practitioner Psychologist, registered with the HCPC.

I trained in EMDR in 2013 and have used EMDR for many years, becoming an EMDR Consultant in 2020. EMDR is a powerful therapy, which can resolve traumatic memories somewhat more quickly than other forms of trauma therapy and set people on a path to a happier more fulfilled life. However, it is vital that the therapist is well trained and supervised in their practice to ensure that they can respond to any destabilisation that may occur during processing and keep the traumatised person within their window of tolerance. Practitioner Psychologists, registered with the HCPC, have a duty to remain up to date with the evidence base and to undertake regular supervision. This means that you can be sure that the person you are seeing is adequately trained and qualified to treat you.

Mindfulness Apps for Self Help

In Chapter 14, I mentioned that there are smartphone apps for mindfulness practice which can make the process easier to learn. The ones that I have tried or had recommended include:

Headspace	https://www.headspace.com/
Calm	https://www.calm.com/
Smiling Mind	https://www.smilingmind.co.uk/
JKZ	https://jonkabat-zinn.com/

There is also the ACT Coach app where you can apply everything we have discussed in this book, including clarifying your values and making those small steps towards a valued future. ACT Coach can be found at https://mobile.va.gov/app/act-coach

These are all available as apps on your smartphone app provider store, but I have pointed you towards their websites to allow you to read more about them before you commit to trying an app. Most of them do have a subscription or cost to download and that is something to take into account. These are just a very few options and if you search your app provider, you will find many, many more possibilities.

Final Words

I hope that by sharing my story I have shown that trauma is a common experience which impacts us in many different and significant ways. Whatever your experience and your ways of coping, you did not ask for it, you did not deserve it and you coped in the best way you knew how at the time. Being human often requires us to face adversity. By learning to sit with our thoughts and feelings mindfully, to turn towards the difficult things and to take small steps in the direction of the life we want to live, we can begin a healing journey towards not just surviving but thriving. Whatever your experience of trauma has been and whatever the impact, I hope that you will find something in this book that is helpful to you as you navigate your journey forwards.

Appendices
Worksheets and Questionnaires

ACE Questionnaire

While you were growing up, during your first 18 years of life:

1. Did a parent or other adult in the household often or very often …

   Swear at you, insult you, put you down or humiliate you?
   or
   Act in a way that made you afraid that you might be physically hurt?
   Yes No   If yes enter 1 _____

2. Did a parent or other adult in the household often or very often …

   Push, grab, slap or throw something at you?
   or
   Ever hit you so hard that you had marks or were injured?
   Yes No   If yes enter 1 _____

3. Did an adult or person at least five years older than you ever …

   Touch or fondle you or have you touch their body in a sexual way?
   or
   Attempt or actually have oral, anal, or vaginal intercourse with you?
   Yes No   If yes enter 1 _____

4. Did you often or very often feel that …

   No one in your family loved you or thought you were important or special?
   or

Appendices

    Your family didn't look out for each other, feel close to each other or support each other?
Yes No   If yes enter 1 _____

5. Did you often or very often feel that …
You didn't have enough to eat, had to wear dirty clothes and had no one to protect you?
or
Your parents were too drunk or high to take care of you or take you to the doctor if you needed it?
Yes No   If yes enter 1 _____

6. Were your parents ever separated or divorced?
Yes No   If yes enter 1 _____

7. Was your mother or stepmother:
Often or very often pushed, grabbed, slapped or had something thrown at her?
or
Sometimes, often, or very often kicked, bitten, hit with a fist or hit with something hard?
or
Ever been repeatedly hit for at least a few minutes or threatened with a gun or knife?
Yes No   If yes enter 1 _____

8. Did you live with anyone who was a problem drinker or alcoholic or who used street drugs?
Yes No   If yes enter 1 _____

9. Was a household member depressed or mentally ill, or did a household member attempt suicide?
Yes No   If yes enter 1 _____

10. Did a household member go to prison?
Yes No   If yes enter 1 _____
Now add up your 'Yes' answers: _____ This is your ACE Score.

Adapted from: http://www.acestudy.org/files/ACE_Score_Calculator.pdf

Four Elements Exercise for Stress Management Adapted from Shapiro (2012)

We cope better with stress when our stress is within manageable levels, so it is helpful to regularly monitor stress and use strategies to reduce stress throughout the day. This exercise contains four brief, self-calming exercises using the sequence of four elements: (1) Earth, (2) Air, (3) Water and (4) Fire.

Four Elements

EARTH: Grounding, Safety in the Present

The first element is earth, it represents the idea of grounding ourselves in the present and noticing that we are safe in the present.

- Take a minute or two to land, to be here now.
- Place both feet on the ground, if you are sitting, feel the chair supporting you.
- Direct your attention outwards and notice three new things that you can see.
- Notice any sounds.
- Notice any smells.

AIR: Breathing for Strength, Balance and Centring

The element of AIR represents a feeling of strength, balance and centring.

- Anxiety is a bit like excitement without oxygen and can result in you stopping breathing effectively.
- If you start noticing your breath and breathing slowly and deeply, your anxiety will decrease.
- So, as you feel the safety of your feet on the ground, take three or four deeper, slower breaths from your stomach to your chest, making sure to breathe all the way out to make room for fresh, energizing air.

- As you breathe out, imagine that you are letting go of some of the stress and breathing it out. Direct your attention inwards, to your centre.
- Notice any positive feelings in your body.

WATER: Calm and Controlled – Switch on the Relaxation Response

Through the element of water, we can switch on the relaxation response and become calm and controlled.

- Notice if you have saliva in your mouth.
- You may have noticed that when you are anxious or stressed, your mouth often feels dry because part of the stress emergency response is to shut off the digestive system. This is controlled by the Sympathetic Nervous System.
- When you start making saliva, you switch on the digestive system again or the para-sympathetic nervous system and the relaxation response.
- This is the reason why people are offered water or tea after a difficult experience.
- You could imagine the taste of a lemon, or something else that makes your mouth 'water' in anticipation. When you make saliva you can optimally control your thoughts and body.
- So, as you continue to feel the safety of your feet on the ground and feel centred as you breathe in and out, direct your attention to making saliva.
- As you continue to feel the safety now of your feet on the ground and feel centred as you breathe in and out and feel calm and in control as you produce more and more saliva, notice any physical sensations in your body and where they are.
- Think about whether the sensations feel good.
- Then, direct your attention to the feeling good in your body and just notice those positive feelings.
- Now think about those three elements of earth, then air and then water. Go with any feelings or images you experience.

FIRE: Light up the Path of Your Imagination

FIRE is the fourth element and is used in this exercise to light up the path of your imagination to access your SAFE PLACE or another resource that is positive for you.

- Think about a place you have been, or can imagine being, that feels very safe or calm. This might be lying on a beach or sitting by a mountain stream.
- Take a moment to think about a place that feels safe, calm or soothing and bring up that image.
- Notice how your body feels as you focus on that image.
- Direct your attention to any positive feelings in your body and enjoy them.
- As you continue to feel the safety now of your feet on the ground and feel centred as you breathe in and out and feel calm and in control as you produce more and more saliva, you can let the fire light the path to your imagination to bring up an image of a place where you feel safe or a memory in which you felt good about yourself.
- Go with that image or memory, and start thinking first about earth, then air, then water and then fire. Go with it and notice any positive sensations in your body.

Breathing Exercises

a. Mindful Breathing
   - Find somewhere quiet and comfortable to sit.
   - Notice, if you are able to, the feeling of your body touching the chair, and your feet on the floor. (Feel free to make any adaptations to the instructions to accommodate any disability issues you may have.)
   - Notice the feeling of your breath entering your nose.
   - Follow the sensations of your breath as it enters your lungs.
   - Notice the movements of your chest and abdomen as the breath fills you up.

Appendices

- Notice that moment as the in-breath stops, there is the briefest of pauses, and the breath turns around and begins to leave the body.
- Notice the release as your body exhales.
- Follow the sensations of the breath as it leaves through your nose or mouth.
- Return to point 3. above and follow the next breath all the way in and all the way out.
- Repeat as often as you like.

b. Box or Square Breathing
- Again, find a quiet and comfortable space if you can.
- Bring your attention to your breathing.
- Visualise a square like the one below and breathe to a count of four around each side of the square, starting at the bottom left hand corner breathing in up the side of the square, holding the breath across the top, breathing out down the other side and holding the breath across the bottom.
- Repeat for several rounds until you feel calmer and more grounded.
- Take a photo on your phone of the square below and refer back to it if you need a visual cue to follow as you practice the exercise.

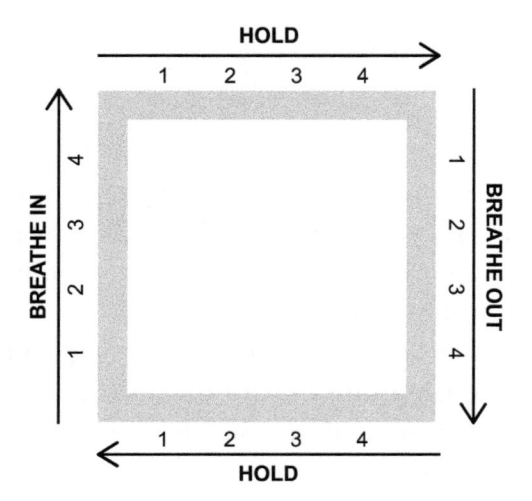

```
              HOLD
         1   2   3   4  →
       ┌─────────────────┐
    ↑  │                 │  ↓
  4 │  │                 │  │ 1
  3 │  │                 │  │ 2   BREATHE OUT
BREATHE IN                  │ 3
  2 │  │                 │  │ 4
  1 │  │                 │
       └─────────────────┘
     ← 1   2   3   4
              HOLD
```

Progressive Muscle Relaxation

- Find a comfortable place either sitting or lying on a chair or bed, or even on the floor on a yoga mat.
- You may wish to close your eyes, but this is not essential.
- Take a few relaxing breaths as described above as you settle into position.
- Bring your attention to the muscles of your head and face, tighten those muscles for two to three seconds, scrunching your eyes and face as you do so and then let the tightness go as you breathe out slowly.
- Move your awareness to the muscles of your neck and shoulders, tighten those muscles for two to three seconds and then let the tightness go on the out-breath.
- Move your attention to the muscles of your arms and hands, tighten the muscles for a couple of seconds and then let the tightness go as you breath out.
- Bring your attention to the muscles of your chest and upper back, tighten them and let them go as you breath out.
- Notice the muscles of your stomach and lower back, tighten and let go, just as before.
- Notice the muscles of your pelvic area and bottom, tighten and let go, just as before.
- Pay attention to the muscles of your legs and feet, tighten them and let them go as you breathe out.
- Just take a few moments to rest in the relaxed state you find yourself in, noticing how your body has softened and let go of tension.

Leaves on the Stream Exercise

- Find a quiet and comfortable place to sit, where you will not be disturbed for a few minutes, maybe up to half an hour, maybe longer. The duration of the exercise is up to you.

- Imagine you are sitting beside a river or a stream with the water flowing gently past, not a raging torrent, and not still waters, something gentle, but moving.
- Picture your surroundings, maybe you are sitting on a comfortable log beside the river's edge, maybe there are trees overhanging the water, dropping the occasional leaf onto the surface of the water, or maybe you can hear birdsong or the rustling of the wind in the trees. Make the scene your own and embellish it however you like.
- Imagine yourself sitting here, enjoying a few moments of peace and tranquillity away from the usual hassles of daily life.
- Always, when we start to relax and take a break like this, our mind starts to get busy, that's normal, don't try to fight it, in fact, do the opposite, accept it and just notice each thought as it pops into your mind.
- As you notice each thought, imagine yourself placing it on a leaf on the surface of the river and watch as it either hangs around or floats away in its own good time.
- It matters not whether these are good thoughts, bad thoughts or somewhere in the middle thoughts, they are just thoughts and can be placed on a leaf to do as they wish.
- Try not to force anything, try to just notice. Don't try to push the thoughts away, place them on a leaf and just be curious.
- If there are no thoughts, just notice that and watch the river flowing by while you listen to the sounds of nature all around. If your mind is a human mind, you can be sure it will start up with random thoughts again very soon.
- Spend as long as you like on this exercise and practice it regularly.

Imagined Resource Figures

- When you face a challenging time dealing with your trauma memories, it can be helpful to imagine having a support team

Appendices

around you. In Chapter 14, I introduced the idea of having your own imagined inner cheerleader. You can expand on this to create any resource figure that you feel you need on your team to deal with your challenges.

- Typically, people need a nurturing figure, a protector figure and a wise guide, but you can really go to town here and create any imagined figure that will provide you with the qualities you need to get through this.
- To give some ideas, people often draw on characters from fiction, creatures from the wild or from fantasy, or they may draw on real people they have come across who exhibit the qualities required.
- Someone who needs courage might conjure up an image of a soldier, a Samurai warrior or a character from their favourite adventure novel.
- Someone who needs compassion may conjure up an image of an ideal mother figure, perhaps from religion or literature.
- Using imagined resources like this can be more difficult if you don't have a strong imagination, so I would suggest using examples such as people you know, or have seen on TV, and just bring them to mind when you need them.
- To develop a resource figure, imagine the qualities you need them to have and think of a person or creature that represents those qualities to you.
- Take a few moments to settle your mind in a quiet, comfortable place. Slow your breathing and relax your body as best you can.
- Try to bring to mind a person or a creature from real life, from fiction, from a movie or from your own imagination who has the quality you desire.
- Think what they would look like. How big are they? How are they dressed? How do they look at you?
- Notice how they move. Are they walking alongside you? Are they floating above you? Are they following you closely?
- Notice what they say and do to support, protect or guide you. How does their voice sound?

- Really take some time to build your character or to recall them if they are from real life, noticing all the aspects of how they look, move and communicate with you.
- Bring this character to mind every time you find yourself struggling, or in need of their particular qualities.

Values Cards

The values in the table below can be copied and cut out to make a set of cards. These can then be sorted until you identify your six most important values for living. These should form the basis for your decision making as you begin to create a life worth living for you.

POWER	SERVICE	KINDNESS
CURIOSITY	LEARNING	LEADERSHIP
FUN	FULFILMENT	TRUST
SUPPORT	FAIRNESS	INTEGRITY
HAPPINESS	JOY	BEAUTY
RESPECT	INNER PEACE	WINNING
SPIRITUALTY	HOPE	INNER STRENGTH
NATURE	NURTURE	PEACE
CREATIVITY	HOME	INDEPENDENCE
ACCEPTANCE	FREEDOM	ADVENTURE
CHALLENGE	HEALTH	WEALTH
FAMILY	CHARITY	FRIENDSHIP
HONESTY	LOVE	COMPASSION
ENCOURAGEMENT	ACHIEVEMENT	LOYALTY
SELF RESPECT	ORDER	STRUCTURE
SECURITY	SAFETY	PATIENCE

(*Continued*)

Appendices

(*Continued*)

CONSISTENCY	WISDOM	PASSION
ADVENTURE	COURAGE	GRATITUDE
SENSUALITY	DIGNITY	CONNECTION
EQUALITY	CARING	RISK

References

American Psychiatric Association (2022) *Diagnostic and Statistical Manual of Mental Disorders: Diagnostic and Statistical Manual of Mental Disorders*, 5th Edition text revision. American Psychiatric Association, Arlington.

Barker MJ & Iantaffi A (2019) *Life Isn't Binary: On Being Both, Beyond, and In-Between.* Jessica Kingsley, London & Philadelphia.

Boon S, Steele K & van der Hart O (2011) *Coping with Trauma Related Dissociation: Skills Training for Patients and Therapists.* WW Norton & Co, New York and London.

Bowlby J (1988). *A Secure Base.* Basic Books, New York.

Brenner J, Pan Z, Mazefsky C, Smith KA & Gabriels R (2018) Behavioural Symptoms of Reported Abuse in Children and Adolescents with Autism Spectrum Disorder in Inpatient Settings. *Journal of Autism and Developmental Disorders 48*(1), 3727–3735. https://doi.org/10.1007/s10803-017-3183-4

Brewin CR & Andrews B (2017) False Memories of Childhood Sexual Abuse. *The Psychologist.* Accessed 24 August 2022 from https://www.bps.org.uk/psychologist/false-memories-childhood-abuse

Carrière R (2013) Healing Trauma, Healing Humanity: Rolf Carrière at TEDx Groningen. https://www.youtube.com/watch?v=CcXqcQecRXo.

Center for Disease Control (CDC) ACES Pyramid. Accessed 24 August 2022 from https://www.cdc.gov/violenceprevention/aces/about.html

Dana D (2018) *The Polyvagal Theory in Therapy Engaging the Rhythm of Regulation.* WW Norton & Co, New York and London.

Felitti, VJ, Anda RF, Nordenberg D, Williamson DF, Spitz AM, Edwards V, Koss MP & Marks JS (1998) Relationship of childhood abuse and household dysfunction to many of the leading causes of death in adults: The Adverse Childhood Experiences (ACE) Study. *American Journal of Preventive Medicine 14*(4), 245–258. https://doi.org/10.1016/S0749-3797(98)00017-8

Fisher J (2017) *Healing the Fragmented Selves of Trauma Survivors.* Routledge, New York and London.

Fisher J (2021) *Transforming the Living Legacy of Trauma a Workbook for Survivors and Therapists.* PESI, Eau Claire.

References

Fraser GA (1991) The Dissociative Table Technique: A Strategy for Working with Ego States in Dissociative Disorders and Ego-State Therapy. *Dissociation* 4(4), 205–213.

Freud S (1896) *The Aetiology of Hysteria*. Accessed 11 February 2022 from https://icpla.edu/wp-content/uploads/2012/10/Freud-S.-Aetiology-of-Hysteria-C.P.-vol.1-1924-p.183-221.pdf

Gilbert P (2010) *The Compassionate Mind*. Constable & Robinson Ltd, London.

Godsi E (1999) *Violence in Society*. Constable & Co Ltd, London.

Gross RD (1992) *Psychology: The Science of Mind and Behaviour*, 2nd Edition. Hodder & Staunton, London.

Harris R (2008) *The Happiness Trap*. Robinson, London.

Harris R (2019) *ACT Made Simple*, 2nd Edition. New Harbinger Publications, Inc, Oakland.

Herman J (1992) *Trauma and Recovery*. Basic Books, New York.

Janoff-Bulman R (1992) *Shattered Assumptions: Towards a New Psychology of Trauma*. Free Press, New York.

Johnstone L & Boyle M with Cromby J, Dillon J, Harper D, Kinderman P, Longden E, Pilgrim D & Rea J. (2018) *The Power Threat Meaning Framework: Towards the Identification of Patterns in Emotional Distress, Unusual Experiences and Troubled or Troubling Behaviour, as an Alternative to Functional Psychiatric Diagnosis*. British Psychological Society, Leicester.

Joseph S, Williams R & Yule W (1993) Changes in Outlook Following Disaster: The Preliminary Development of a Measure to Assess Positive and Negative Responses. *Journal of Traumatic Stress* 6(2), 271–279.

Kabat-Zinn J (1996) *Full Catastrophe Living: How to Cope with Stress, Pain and Illness Using Mindfulness Meditation*. Little Brown Book Group, London.

King R (2010) Commentary: Complex Post traumatic Stress Disorder: Implications for individuals with Autism Spectrum Disorders – Part I. *Journal on Developmental Disabilities* 16, 91–100.

King R & Desaulnier CL (2011) Commentary: Complex Post Traumatic Stress Disorder: Implications for Individuals with Autism Spectrum Disorders – Part II. *Journal on Developmental Disabilities* 17, 47–59.

Levine PA (1997) *Waking the Tiger – Healing Trauma*. North Atlantic Books, Berkeley.

Luoma JB, Hayes SC & Walser R (2007) *Learning ACT An Acceptance and Commitment Therapy Skills Training Manual for Therapists*. New Harbinger Publications Inc, Oakland.

Martell CR, Addis ME & Jacobson NS (2013) *Behavioural Activation for Depression: A Clinician's Guide*. 1st Edition. The Guidlford Press, Guildford.

Maslow AH (1943) A Theory of Human Motivation. *Psychological Review* 50(4), 370–396.

Maté G (2008) *In the Realm of Hungry Ghosts*. Vintage Canada.

References

Mehtar M & Mukaddes NM (2011) Posttraumatic Stress Disorder in individuals with diagnosis of Autism Spectrum Disorders. *Research in Autism Spectrum Disorders 5*, 539–546.

NICE Guideline Post-traumatic stress disorder [NG116] Published: 05 December 2018. Accessed 9 February 2022 from https://www.nice.org.uk/guidance/ng116/chapter/Context

Ogden P, Minton K, Pain C, Siegel DJ & van der Kolk BA (2006) *Trauma and the Body: A Sensorimotor Approach to Psychotherapy*. W.W. Norton & Co, New York and London.

Oliver M (1996) *Understanding Disability from Theory to Practice*. Macmillan Press, London.

Paulsen S (2017) *When There Are No Words: Repairing Early Trauma and Neglect from the Attachment Period with EMDR Therapy*. Bainbridge Institute for Integrative Psychology, Bainbridge Island, WA.

Perry BD & Szalavitz M (2017) *The Boy Who Was Raised as a Dog, 3rd Edition: And Other Stories from a Child Psychiatrist's Notebook--What Traumatized Children Can Teach Us About Loss, Love, and Healing*. Basic Books, New York.

Pope KS (1996) Memory, Abuse, and Science: Questioning Claims About the False Memory Syndrome Epidemic. *American Psychologist 51*(9), 957–974.

Porges SW (2009) The Polyvagal Theory: New Insights into Adaptive Reactions of the Autonomic Nervous System. *Cleveland Clinic Journal of Medicine 76*(4 suppl 2), S86–S90.

Rothschild B (2000) *The Body Remembers: The Psychophysiology of Trauma and Trauma Treatment*. W.W. Norton & Company Inc, New York.

Sacks O (1985) *The Man Who Mistook His Wife for a Hat*. Summit Books, New York.

Sacks O (1989) *Seeing Voices: a Journey into the World of the Deaf*. University of California Press, Berkeley.

Sacks O (1990) *Awakenings*. Harper Perennial, New York.

Sacks O (1995) *An Anthropologist on Mars*. Knopf, New York.

Shapiro E (2012) – 4 Elements Exercise. *Journal of EMDR Practice and Research 1*(2), 113–115

Shapiro F (1990; revised 2021) *EMDR Therapy Basic Training Manual*. EMDR Institute Inc, Watsonville.

Shapiro F (2018) *Eye Movement Desensitization and Reprocessing (EMDR) Therapy*, 3rd Edition. Guildford Publications, New York.

Siegal D (2002) *The Developing Mind: How Relationships and the Brain Interact to Shape Who We Are*. Guildford Press, New York.

Spring C (2019) *Unshame: Healing Trauma Based Shame Through Psychotherapy*. Carolyn Spring Publishing, Huntingdon.

References

Stack A & Lucyshin J (2021) Chapter 5: Trauma in Individuals with Autism Spectrum Disorder: An Empirically Informed Model of Assessment and Intervention to Address the Effects of Traumatic Events. In FR Volkmar et al. (Eds.) *Handbook of Autism Spectrum Disorder and the Law.* Springer Nature, Switzerland, 97–126.

Van der Kolk B (2015) *The Body Keeps the Score.* Penguin Random House, New York.

Waft YL (2006) (unpublished thesis, University of Leeds Library) Posttraumatic Growth in People Disabled by Traumatic Illness or Injury.

World Health Organisation (2022) ICD-11: International classification of diseases (11th revision). https://icd.who.int/.